DIG PREGNANCY, BIRTH, & BABY

A Conscious & Empowered Approach
to Prenatal & Postnatal Yoga

by Sue Elkind
digpregnancy.com
email: sue@digyoga.com

Cover photo: Art Streiber/AUGUST
Yoga illustrations: Sue Elkind
Book layout: Sue Elkind & Lynnell Koser
Editing: Clare Brown, Mariel Freeman, Dana Covello

Note: It is advisable for all pregnant women to consult with their physician before undertaking any
exercise program. This book is not intended as a substitute for professional medical care.

*For my husband, Naime Jezzeny who teaches me
everyday the importance of being true to oneself,
and our two boys Luca and Milo who through my
pregnancies ignited my passion for prenatal yoga.*

This workbook is a labor of love, one that Sue has put together over the past fourteen years. Her vibrancy, well-honed teaching skills, and sensitivity to individual needs are earmarks of Sue's teaching — and ones that captured my heart as her yoga student.

The information in this book is the result of passionate research and practical applications with pregnant women throughout the world as well as intensely personal observations based on her own experiences of pregnancy with her beloved sons, Luca and Milo.

Dr. Mae Sakharov, Ed. D
Educational consultant to ABC "20/20"

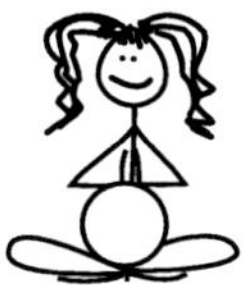

Prenatal Lullaby
SHANTI MANTRA
For harmonious relationships

Saha navavatu
Saha nau bhunaktu
Saha viryam karavavahai
Tejasvi navadhitamastu
Ma vidvishavahai
Om Shanti Shanti Shantih

May both of us together be protected
May both of us together be nourished
May we work together with great energy
May our study together be brilliant and effective
May we not dispute with each other
Om Peace Peace Peace

* Chanting is a beautiful way to connect
mother and baby throughout pregnancy – the baby
delights in hearing the mother's voice.

This invocation can be offered as a prenatal lullaby
and often has a calming effect on the baby after birth.

TABLE OF CONTENTS

REFLECTIONS BY SIANNA SHERMAN

We are all carried in the womb of the Great Mother, all men and all women. Birth requires gestation in the warm flowing waters of the Goddess where our heartbeat is one with our mother. The months from conception to our first breath of air are a time of sanctuary, preparing us for the immense journey ahead as a human being on the planet. Each of us holds the embodied memories of these most sublime months living within our mother, where we first listen to her voice and learn to make connections from the inside out.

The life of a woman is filled with pulsating cycles and rhythmic attunement with all of nature and especially the moon. Every woman undergoes initiations, whether consciously or not, through the 3 great phases of her life: Maiden, Mother, and Wise Woman. One symbol that has long been revered is the Triple Spiral, which helps a woman to recognize her own flowing nature through the secret passageways of time as she flowers open and turns within.

In the years of the Mother, a woman may choose to usher life forth through her own womb. Some women do not make this particular choice, yet they are still Mothers too. They are mothers of the planet, mothers of the creative life force energy that surges through them, and mothers who hold the space of awakening for the benefit of all beings.

Just as all women are mothers, all women are also warriors. We are warriors of love, remembrance and living wisdom. Women who give physical birth must summon forth their highest bravery and require the support of other women to stand by their side in a lineage of sisterhood that stretches through time. This book is for all women. Women who will go through pregnancy and childbirth and women who wish to support their sisters through this extraordinary gateway.

Sue Elkind is a yogini, mother and priestess of modern-day wisdom born through her own experience and through her many years of training with some of the most renowned teachers in the great tradition of yoga. In this book, Sue calls forth the sacredness of the journey from pre-conception to the fourth trimester where the mother embraces her child in her arms. The entire cycle welcomes a time of listening, alignment and skillful action. Sue's accessible and loving book offers practical information so every mother can prepare the way with intelligent, well-informed choices.

This book is one of the most important resources for pregnancy and offers a full scope of yoga practices to support the mother through her journey. Every woman will feel the living, breathing wisdom of this book and the victorious call of her own courage that the journey requires for life to be born again and again.

Victory to the Mother! Salutations to the Goddess in all Women! Jaya Mataji!
Sianna Sherman (San Francisco, California, 2012)

FOREWORD   BY DOUGLAS BROOKS

Yoga invites us to engage deeply, to create connections, and to affirm wholly the fullness of our lives. And what gift in life presents a greater opportunity for yoga or a more profound offering of Grace than the experience of pregnancy?

The tradition of women caring for women extends deeply into the ancient yogas, and in Tantra we learn of the woman-sage Lopamudra. Lopamudra is the guardian of the life-giving inner waters; the presence of Grace holding purity within; and the teacher of midwives, yoginis, and all who seek the subtle powers of the Shakti's most receptive energies during prenatal care. Tradition says that Lopamudra was a princess born as a boon to the King of Kavera granted to him by none other than grandfather Creator Brahma. After she was married to the great sage Agastya, the princess took the form of water within her husband's sacred vessel. Once Agastya asked his yogic student to carry this vessel, but he could not bear its weight. And so the water that was Lopamudra spilt, rushing forth as the river Kaveri. When King Kavera bathed in this now-famous south Indian river that began as none other than his daughter's own form, he experienced his own liberation. And so it is that all who step into Lopamudra's subtle presence as the life-holding waters are too born to experience their freedom. What a story! But with a little Tantric ingenuity, we can further savor its sweetness.

Lopamudra's name means the seal or imprint (mudra) of interruption or sometimes even injury (lopa). As a child grows in the womb so this gift "interrupts" the usual patterns of life and creates its own imprint from inside out. Giving birth is a perfect, blessed "injury" creating the most auspicious gift we might ever receive. In the meantime, a baby floats and swims in its mother, the sacred vessel, protected there by love through partnership, and with the help of the mother's companions, shares her yogic journey. When a child is ready to spill forth into the world, from the inner waters of grace, she or he will come to purify, to bless, and even to liberate all who have come before as well as those who follow. Every mother becomes Lopamudra, that vessel of the sacred, the waters within her being a gift of Grace to the emergent life she holds, and her yoga the process by which to engage fully in the offerings of pregnancy and birth.

With Sue Elkind as your guide and the principles of yoga to lead the way, I know you are in the best of hands to make or advise others in this journey. For pregnant women, with the practices of yoga, you will feel even more deeply the imprint of that precious soul you carry within as the expression of your body's grace. May these teachings of yoga inspire your heart and empower your body! May the ancient teachings become present, enriching, and real in your experience of pregnancy, birth, and motherhood! I know this book will be a gift and a blessing, nothing less than another form of Lopamudra spilling forth her blessings and teachings, for once again the ancient sage presents herself in your own experience of yoga. Jaya Lopamudra the Sage! Jaya Mataji, the Auspicious Mother!

Douglas Brooks (Bristol, New York, 2009)

MY STORY

My interest in prenatal yoga developed shortly after I began teaching yoga in the early 1990's. During one of my first public classes, I encountered a pregnant student who was in obvious need of extra assistance. Trying not to panic, I instinctively gave her as many props as I could find to help her modify her practice and stayed close by to remind her to breathe! After the session, I called a seasoned prenatal yoga teacher and friend, Susan Swan, to consult about what I had done. First she assured me that I did not do anything wrong or harmful. She then offered me some useful advice based on her wisdom and personal experiences in pregnancy and prenatal yoga. From that first experience, I was truly inspired to see how yoga and the state of pregnancy were deeply connected. I continued to seek out prenatal trainings over the next several years, fortunate to be in Los Angeles where prenatal yoga was flourishing. There was an abundance of great inspiration, particularly the community woven together by Gurmukh Khalsa. What I found interesting was how different each prenatal yoga class was — depending on the teacher and their school of influence. When I became pregnant and decided to teach prenatal yoga, I used this multitude of resources I had gathered to help inspire my own voice to bloom.

My hope with this book is that teachers, students, and others interested in the connection between pregnancy and yoga will gain a deeper understanding of the many gifts that prenatal and postnatal yoga offer to support pregnancy, birth, and beyond. A teacher trained to work with the specific conditions of the pregnant body — including the ability to encourage a student to really trust in her experience, can greatly help to create a safe, healthy, and empowering prenatal and postnatal yoga practice.

My greatest source of prenatal wisdom has undoubtedly come from having two very different pregnancies and birth experiences. Although both were homebirths, my first pregnancy was much more conventional than the second. Being cautious after already having had a miscarriage, I listened diligently to my doctor and the spiritual guidance of my cherished doula Anna Verwaal (a doula is often translated as "mother's mother" and is there to support the mother during the birth process). My beloved yoga teachers offered wonderful insight into my personal practice and the best gift of all — the confidence to be my own teacher and explore my pregnancy and practice from a deep inner wisdom.

While I initially thought a conventional hospital birth would be my route, about four weeks before my first son, Luca, was born, I found a new house more suitable to do a home birth and switched to a midwife. When the first real contractions started, I felt that I had prepared as best as possible. What I did not expect was that my labor would last thirty-two hours. I was fully dilated when my water finally broke in the bathtub. My midwife noticed the amniotic fluid contained meconium (a thick, tar-like stool that a baby typically releases after he or she is born). Luca had a bowel movement while still in the womb, which meant there was a chance he could aspirate meconium into his lungs upon arrival. Although this situation is fairly common, it was nonetheless frightening. Our pediatrician, Jay Gordon, came rushing to the house hoping to avoid taking Luca to the hospital. After listening to his lungs for a solid hour, everyone agreed it was not worth the risk. Luca spent the first week of his life in neo-natal intensive care with tubes up his nose to help him breathe and had continuous monitoring for infection. Looking back, Luca and I had extraordinary moments together the first hour of his life, and I was fortunate to avoid the higher risk of a c-section surgery, a standard procedure when meconium is detected. Even though my home birth did not go according to my plan, I had an important revelation: birth is not just about a mother's wishes and plans. Luca's birth wasn't just my dance.

My second son, Milo, on the other hand, arrived while I was in a very deep state of meditation — without even pushing — in a truly bucolic birth in the comforts of our dimly lit bedroom. Both my husband Naime and I were astonished at the beauty and bliss of Milo's sweet entrance into the world and bathed for hours in the afterglow. Reflecting on this pregnancy, I barely had any intervention, choosing instead to use a stethoscope when possible and the skillful hands of my midwives, Shelly Girard and Seannie Gibson. I stayed 'tuned in' through regular meditation and trusted what I heard inwardly with even greater sensitivity and awareness. My confidence to do this was bolstered immensely by having both the strength and support of my midwives who continuously guided me, along with my family and friends standing close by.

Looking back at my birth experiences, I realize how important it is for a pregnant woman to be surrounded by loving, supportive, and understanding friends. Without the emotional security of a kula (community of like-minded hearts), it is much harder to relax and trust our inherent wisdom. This is one of the main reasons why I feel prenatal yoga classes, if available, are such a powerful and indispensable part of a woman's pregnancy for both experienced practitioners and those new to yoga.

THE INNER WISDOM OF YOGA IN PREGNANCY

From one creative Universal force, all of life emerges. Divine energy takes the form of everything manifest and unseen — expanding, contracting, and radiating from this light of existence. Each one of us is an expression of this Supreme Consciousness, whose innate nature is love and joy. Yoga strengthens this awareness and enables us to step fully into ourselves — body, mind, and heart. As we learn to trust in this universal connection and recognize how deeply supported we are, we can more freely let go of fears and experience our lives with greater understanding, compassion, and joy.

Pregnancy offers a woman the opportunity to tap into and participate in the creative energy of the Universe. The threshold into motherhood is an extremely powerful time of heightened sensitivity and growth on multiple levels. From a yogic perspective, pregnancy is a sacred time for a woman to discover her own intuitive strength and nurture the creative feminine power within. For many women, this inner shift of awareness occurs naturally. Instinctually, the body lures the mind inward to notice and care for all the physical, emotional, and hormonal changes beginning to occur. As the fetus begins to grow, a powerful maternal urge to nurture and protect often naturally ignites. Practicing yoga enhances and empowers a woman's experience of pregnancy and birth on all levels — physically, emotionally, and spiritually. Through the ever-unfolding gifts of yoga, the process of giving birth becomes not only an invitation to deepen one's innermost connection to the Universe, but also a celebration of the profound, regenerative, and sacred power each woman holds.

Pregnancy and birth are both singularly extraordinary and universally common. Everyone alive on this planet is united in the commonality that they must be 'born' to get here — yet throughout the world, birth experiences range from the most primitive and natural, to the most scheduled and scientific. We are both cultural and natural beings, regardless of how we arrived on this planet. The power to think and reason does not make us any less connected to nature — although sometimes it is our own minds that get in the way of that understanding. Practicing yoga while pregnant invites a woman to pulsate between her natural and cultural sides. Some women more easily recognize the cultured side of pregnancy — embracing their noted glow and outer beauty. However it is equally essential for a pregnant woman to draw into her innermost primal essence — not only as a means to uncover and transform any deep-seated fears, but also to strengthen her resolve and recognize that the power to create life is inherent. Through the process of diving inward, a woman can experience her divine nature more authentically, allowing her to see more beauty and interconnectedness in the world.

When a woman has the courage to face the darkness of her pregnancy head on, she discovers that beneath the fear and discomfort is the support of the primordial Goddess, Kali. Often depicted as pure blackness, Kali is the first Hindu Goddess to take form. She is sometimes known as the original mother, though she is nothing like you would expect a mother to be! She is radical, wild, and ferocious, and while she loves to stretch us to our outer boundaries, her intention is always to take us deeper into our hearts to feel her unconditional love. When a woman is going through labor, she must learn to trust her own Kali-like nature and release any inhibitions around her pregnancy and the process of giving birth. If she is able to step fully into her experience, before accepting or denying it, she will feel the nurturing roar of Kali and discover even more strength available within her — empowering her birth and preparing her for motherhood. It is also the embrace of Kali that allows a woman to move forward when her labor takes an unplanned course.

The pulsation of pregnancy also calls for a woman to seek the wisdom and generosity of others and to appreciate the beauty of her outer environment. All of the many ways a woman can enjoy and share her pregnancy with the world are reflected in the refined, cultured energy of the Goddess Shri. She becomes the expression of all that is beautiful and sacred about being pregnant. A woman taps into Shri when she chooses to listen to her body each day and comes from a place of love, honor, and respect for herself and the miracle of life growing within.

In addition to connecting to the power and the beauty of the goddess within, it is helpful for a pregnant woman to remember she is not alone in the birth process. It greatly benefits a woman to surround herself with a competent and loving team of support, so she can relax and trust them to guide her to the safest delivery possible. In particular, just being in the company of other pregnant women in prenatal yoga classes may create an instant sense of community — a place for information, understanding, and friendship.

PLANNING FOR PREGNANCY

There's a funny thing that happens to many women somewhere between their mid 20's, 30's, and 40's. Thoughts may begin to creep in about babies, and as much as the modern woman may want to deny them, the urge is strong. In many ways, it is the most natural instinct a woman can have. It's hormonal. It's evolutionary. Once the seed is planted, every thought begins to water that idea into more possibility — and ultimately, for some, into motherhood.

A woman enters her pregnancy in myriad ways. Whether it is planned and conventional, unconventional or unexpected, Mother Nature has no 'moral' preference regarding conception. The simple, yet complex scientific dance of sperm penetrating egg has yielded results for eons. While a woman cannot control the intricacies during that time of conception or her pregnancy, there are some helpful things she can do beforehand to ensure a healthier experience from preconception through childbirth.

The first thing she can do is slow down and examine her current life. If work responsibilities are piling up and each day ends in stress, adding a child to the mix isn't going to make it easier. As hard as it may be, creating more space now, before pregnancy, is an important step in preparing for motherhood — physically, mentally, and emotionally. During both of my pregnancies, I found taking regular walks in nature and routinely having nourishing, romantic meals with Naime helped to alleviate stress and restore deeper commitments to creating a family.

Good physical health should be a priority before conceiving. Getting a thorough doctor's examination, for both the woman and man, can help detect and/or ward off any unwanted problems or conditions (i.e checking health of sperm, screening for sexually transmitted diseases). A woman should find an OB/GYN with whom she is comfortable and have a full check-up, including a pap smear and blood work. With her doctor's advice, she may consider taking prenatal supplements (including folic acid to prevent neural tube defects) and start paying closer attention to her diet. I recommend buying organic food and avoiding chemicals, pesticides, and genetically modified foods as much as possible, as well as drinking filtered water to avoid lead, excess chlorine, metals, and synthetic hormones. To improve her overall health and in preparation for the extra resources needed for the healthy development of a baby, a woman can increase certain foods such as organic fresh produce; whole grain foods; organic chicken, fish, and eggs; and natural live yogurt. Fortunately, there are many books and web sites that offer nutrition for preconception and pregnancy as well as ways to maintain a healthy balanced diet for life (see the Additional Resources section beginning on page 110).

A consistent yoga practice prior to conception will help cultivate a deeper sense of awareness and attune a woman's body to its natural rhythms. It will also strengthen and open the body, preparing it for childbirth. Yoga time should include breath work and meditation. Using visualizations of pregnancy and motherhood can help... energy follows intention.

It is important for a woman to remember there is no 'right' way to be pregnant or to give birth. Just as each person is unique in their own way, so too is every pregnancy unique, deeply personal, and cloaked in majesty. Yoga teaches us to celebrate both our diversity and commonality. It invites us to affirm the particular way in which the Divine has taken form as our individual experience and the universal process of childbirth. Oftentimes, a woman feels she has failed if her ideas around getting pregnant, or even childbirth, do not go according to her plan. Yoga teaches a woman to let go of expectations and to remember the baby too is part of the process and may have a different plan.

PREGNANCY HURDLES: MISCARRIAGE AND INFERTILITY

I can honestly say that I never had the urge to have a baby before getting pregnant. The closest I had come to that mothering instinct was 'birthing' a new yoga studio in Los Angeles, which I poured my heart and soul into making happen. To my surprise, only weeks into the studio opening, Naime and I discovered we were going to have a 'real' baby. I felt overwhelmed to say the least. When we finally both got over the shock and we contemplated our future together as a family, we actually discovered a deep joy arising. Then, almost nine weeks into the pregnancy, I had a miscarriage. It was more of a shocker than getting pregnant. Being a health-conscious yoga teacher, the possibility never entered my mind. We grieved the loss, as expected, but also recognized the spark was still present within us. The seed had been planted and we felt a definite shift into a deeper commitment to our relationship. I owe so much of my recovery from miscarriage to my regular yoga and meditation practice. Asana helped me to physically regain strength more efficiently, while meditation aided my emotional state — helping me stay connected to the little soul I knew would still someday join us.

We spent the next twelve months 'keeping the door open' — with the intention to get pregnant with grace and ease. I kept my prenatal supplements going with the doctor's advice and visualized our family in my meditations. We decided to get married and shortly after, to our sweet delight, discovered we were pregnant. We were infinitely more prepared for our pregnancy having that year between miscarriage and conception. Although it doesn't always work out that way, for us having that time helped us more fully 'conceive' the life we wanted to create.

Miscarriage is always a possibility, particularly in early stages of pregnancy. That is why during the first trimester some women choose to contain the news of the secret life growing within. Fifteen percent of known pregnancies end in miscarriage, according to the American College of Obstetricians and Gynecologists (ACOG), and the majority of them happen in the first trimester. When a woman discovers she has had a miscarriage, it is often wrought with feelings of guilt as she wonders what she might have done to cause it. The majority of the time, it is just the way Mother Nature corrects herself. Grieving the loss of the fetus is healthy and important, and may create an even greater certainty within a woman about her desire to become a mother. There have been many cases of healthy births after even as many as four miscarriages beforehand.

The recovery after a miscarriage is different for every woman. In general, the later the pregnancy loss, the greater the period of physical recovery. Whether a woman miscarries naturally or surgically, by dilation and curettage (D&C), may also impact the healing process. The latter (surgically) takes a considerably shorter time to recover from — averaging around two weeks for bleeding to fully subside and hormone-induced mood swings to even out. Early pregnancy miscarriage resembles light to heavy menstrual bleeding and cramps, which is why some women do not realize they are having one. I recommend waiting until after all heavy bleeding has stopped before a woman returns to her regular yoga practice (as well as getting approval from her doctor). She should also avoid ALL inversions (even down dog) until she has completely recovered. There are some helpful yoga poses to do at home that may provide relief from cramping and mood swings. Seated forward bends like upavista konasana and reclining gentle twists, both with a bolster propped up underneath the belly, may provide comfort.

The emotional recovery is another story altogether and could take substantially longer, especially considering no two people grieve in the same way. Pranayama (see the breathing exercises beginning on page 22) and meditation are both helpful tools in supporting a woman throughout her personal journey towards healing. A regular yoga routine, once the physical body has recovered, will also help to keep her energy levels up and gradually uplift her spirits.

The following is a list of contemplations and affirmations to include in a meditation practice in the event of a miscarriage:

> 'I understand this was just Mother Nature's way, and I am not at fault.'
> 'I am hopeful the perfect soul will be back again soon.'
> 'My body is healing as it should and has the wisdom to create life.'
> 'I trust that all is well and happening in its perfect time.'

If a couple is having difficulty conceiving, both parties should seek medical attention to better understand what, if any, physical limitations are present. A woman should discontinue taking birth control pills (or remove her IUD, if applicable) for a solid three months before trying to conceive to give her body a chance to readjust and restore normal metabolic functions. Caffeine, alcohol, and smoking may increase the risk of miscarriage and birth defects and should be minimized or avoided. To ensure she is getting the necessary vitamins and minerals, a woman should consider taking prenatal vitamins (including folic acid), and if she is a strict vegetarian, consult with a nutritionist to make sure certain foods, like soy, are not affecting her fertility.

In addition to getting medical advice (The Center for Disease Control and Prevention is a good resource: www.cdc.gov/reproductivehealth/infertility/), a woman can try treating infertility using therapeutic applications of yoga. The first thing an experienced yoga teacher should look for is whether a woman's energy is 'up-rooted.' Stress, of any kind, is a big reason for this disruption in the natural, downward flow of energy (apana vayu). Overworking, excessively wearing high heels, or even losing touch with one's 'softer' feminine side, can all cause this type of aggravation. Depending on where a woman holds her stress, her legs, pelvis, and/or back muscles can over tighten and actually cause a lift or shift in the inner organs — including the ovaries. Once the ovaries are even slightly agitated, a woman's ability to conceive may become greatly reduced.

The femurs (upper leg bones) will usually shift forward in the hip socket with this type of disruption of apana vayu. A simple way to check a woman's state is to look at her legs while she's lying down on the floor (on her back with her legs straight.) If her legs are lifted up away from the floor (even when you actively have her move them down) the femurs are too far forward. While supine, rooting the femur bones down (towards the hamstrings) will help to re-align the energy flows and optimally align the inner organs. Using biomechanical principles of yoga, a woman with uprooted femurs should emphasize turning the inner edges of her feet, legs, and pelvis 'in,' moving them 'back,' and even widening them 'apart' before scooping her tailbone. The infertility yoga sequence beginning on page 100 focuses on the poses that support the rooting of femurs to help those who may experience difficulty conceiving.

AN INTRODUCTION TO YOGA PHILOSOPHY

One of the most memorable things I learned as a yoga teacher was to look for the beauty in my students before adjusting their posture. I was trained to see the body as a temple that houses Divine energy and to make particular physical, therapeutic adjustments to enhance the light that was already present within the body. This life-affirming attitude continues to inspire every aspect of my teaching and helps to set the tone in my classes for students to step more fully into their hearts. When I began to teach prenatal yoga, it was seamless how complementary this philosophy was to pregnancy and how truly supportive it could be to help women more confidently step into their potential and celebrate their journey.

The study of yoga is as vast as the ocean, so I will only briefly explain the historical context from which this life-affirming philosophy originates. There are three main schools or 'streams' of yoga, which have the following distinct characteristics:

CLASSICAL YOGA

Classical Yoga appears around the 2nd century, and includes within its umbrella the famous aphorisms known as The Yoga Sutras of Patanjali. This school subscribes to a 'dualist' philosophy that separates Supreme Consciousness (Purusha) as distinctively separate from you and everything in the relative world (Prakriti).

ADVAITA VEDANTA

Following Classical Yoga, the next school to emerge was Advaita Vedanta, around the 8th century, which shifts from the dualist paradigm to a non-dual belief that spirit and matter are not different. This philosophy believes that difference in this material universe is just an illusion (maya) and that recognition of this identity (that we are all really One) leads one to liberation.

TANTRA

The Tantra began around the 7th century, and takes the premise that everything in life is the pulsation (spanda) of Supreme Consciousness (Shiva) and all things manifest (Shakti). It is also non-dual, meaning the 'creator' (the Universe, God, the Divine, etc.) is not separate from the 'creation' (all things manifest--your body, mind, the world). Rather, it welcomes diversity and honors the body and the mind as sacred vessels through which we can discover our true nature and celebrate our lives as a gift of Grace.

THE POWER OF SHAKTI

The Sanskrit word Shakti literally means power. Shakti is described as the manifest form of Consciousness, which includes every thought, feeling, articulation and creation imaginable. Shakti is also referred to as the Great (Maha) Goddess who literally is dancing with you, co-mingled into your every breath. Your inhalations are a gift of her Grace, which is none other than her exhalation. As you exhale, she is drawing in her inhalation. Regardless of your acknowledgement of her, she stays with you until your very last breath; yet, she also delights in your recognition of her.

A woman can truly soar in her pregnancy and birth if she allows herself to trust in this most intimate relationship with the Goddess within. Seeking the wisdom of her own body's intelligence, a woman is able to connect more deeply to the power of her heart, mind and body and recognize this as a manifestation of Shakti. The power of the heart is known as Iccha Shakti, the power of the mind is Jnana Shakti and the power of the body is Kriya Shakti.

ICCHA SHAKTI

Iccha Shakti is defined as the power of the heart's intention. It is one's desire and will, lighting the way as a force behind every action and expression. This power is the place from which a pregnant woman can begin to honor herself as a Goddess. It invites her to recognize the miracle of life growing within and reminds her to see the process of pregnancy and birth — in whatever form it takes — as Sacred.

During every trimester, contemplating the power of Iccha Shakti is a way for a pregnant woman to reflect on the strength of her deepest emotions, and regardless of how she may feel physically on any given day, remember she has the resources within to uplift herself spiritually and emotionally. Connecting to the breath and practicing prenatal yoga are both excellent tools to aid her in her process.

PRENATAL CONTEMPLATIONS:
What qualities of the heart am I feeling today?
What is motivating me in my practice?
Are my thoughts/emotions in alignment with my highest intention?
Am I open to whatever course my pregnancy and labor may take?

JNANA SHAKTI

Jnana Shakti is defined as the mindful awareness of how parts of the body, mind and spirit are connected. It refers to the way in which a pregnant woman consciously listens to what her body and baby are telling her, while she seeks the outside knowledge necessary to maintain good health. Jnana Shakti is at play when a woman chooses to infuse every movement with breath and love, respecting the process of pregnancy as a daily exploration filled with both mystery and wonder.

Contemplating the power of Jnana Shakti, a woman learns to trust her inner guidance and intuition, courageously asking the questions necessary to promote optimal health and well-being for herself and her baby.

> PRENATAL CONTEMPLATIONS:
> How is my body changing today?
> How can I best support these changes?
> What can I do to honor myself and the baby more today?
> What else can I do to support the birth of my baby?

KRIYA SHAKTI

Kriya Shakti is defined as the powerful action of the body. It is the natural energetic pulsation of the body that is both stabilizing (engaging, contracting) and freeing (expanding). It invites a woman to move purposefully through pregnancy, balancing the energy in her body in order to both strengthen and protect herself and baby, while simultaneously allowing space for expansion and growth.

By maintaining good muscular engagement and joint stabilization while practicing yoga, the natural tendencies of the hormone relaxin to open the body become more balanced. As a woman progresses in her pregnancy, she has the opportunity to integrate all that she has learned into the actions of birthing her baby and stepping more gracefully into motherhood.

> PRENATAL CONTEMPLATIONS:
> Have I been using the right amount of effort in my practice today?
> Have I spent time nurturing/taking care of myself?
> Have I given proper attention to my growing baby?
> Have I let others help me?

THE ESSENTIALS OF A HEALTHY PRENATAL YOGA PRACTICE

BREATH

The breath is the Divine's manifestation into each of us. It is the very thing that connects us all in life, and yet each of us has our own experience of it. Pregnancy is the only time when two heartbeats (mother and child) share one breath. Through the breath, the mother can consciously communicate her innermost feelings to her baby. The more lovingly a woman brings her awareness to the breath, the more it naturally expands and relaxes into both her and her baby.

Cultivating a yogic breath called '*ujjayi*' is a powerful tool to help a woman calm the mind and relax the body throughout her pregnancy and in the early stages of labor. *Ujjayi* breathing can be done by tightening the glottis muscles in the back of the throat and making a whisper-like sound on both inhalation and exhalation. As active labor progresses, staying attuned to the breath will help a woman remain more deeply in her 'primal zone' — allowing the proper hormones to be released, the cervix to naturally dilate, and stronger contractions to occur that ultimately support delivery. The breath becomes a wonderful companion for a woman to feel less tension mentally and physically and can support her in fully participating (and enjoying!) the birth process.

Pranayama (expanding the breath through various breathing exercises) is a great way for a woman to build concentration, focus the mind, and connect more fully to her baby. The word '*prana*' literally means life force and is the key to all health and wellbeing. *Prana* is also described as the divine Goddess Shakti. Rather than controlling *prana* (the Goddess), we learn to dance with her. The more a woman can connect to the pulsations of Shakti, the more energy, clarity, and peace she will feel during pregnancy, and the more she will experience her labor with greater understanding.

Breathing Exercises

Slow *Ujjayi* Breathing — Expand the breath slowly and evenly, cultivating a rich smooth sound. Begin to put a count to the inhalation. Start with four and increase the count as necessary (when easy). Make sure the beginning and the end of each inhalation is even, rather than drawing in more breath quickly and tapering off at the end. Then, just as deeply and smoothly, exhale the breath for the same count as the inhalation. It is important to remember not to hold the breath.

Belly Breathing — On the inhalation, take a deep diaphragmatic breath and fill the belly completely. On the exhalation, draw the belly backward toward the spine until the lumbar feels a slight lengthening. Because this breath offers maximum amounts of oxygen to mother and baby, a pregnant woman may feel light-headed at first and might need to cut back to a more shallow belly breath until she can perform the exercise without this side-effect. Belly breathing will help to strengthen the transverse abdominals, which support the lower back and help keep the abdominals from over-separating.

Alternate Nostril Breathing — Raising the right hand, place the thumb to the right nostril, closing off that side of the nose. Inhale only into the left nostril slowly and evenly. Then closing the left nostril with the ring finger and pinky, exhale only out of the right nostril. Continue to alternate right and left sides in this same way for four to eight rounds and then release the hand and breathe naturally a few breaths. Do not hold or retain the breath.

Sitali **Breath** — This is a sipping breath that is done by breathing through a curled tongue (long sides fold towards each other, creating a tube-like shape) on the inhalation, and then closing the mouth and exhaling through the nostrils. It is especially helpful to do when a woman is hot; the inhalation has a cooling quality when drawn in this way. For tongues that do not curl, the inhalation can be done by gently placing the teeth on top of the tip of the tongue while sipping the breath in lightly.

Grounding Breath — Take a slow deep inhalation through the nose, then exhale through the mouth making a whispering 'ha' sound. This breath also has a cooling quality and helps to ground a woman's energy at the end of her yoga practice, or just simply to relieve stress. Use when needed. Even just three slow breaths can make a difference!

Note: Pregnant women should **NEVER** hold their breath while practicing *pranayama*.

ASANA

Understanding the biomechanics of asana is a therapeutic way for prenatal yoga students to experience the fullest expression of their bodies, minds, and hearts. Along with the utilization of the breath in each asana, there are several other essential 'ingredients' that support cultivating a deeper awareness in one's yoga practice. These include Foundation, General Form, Primary Energy Flows and Refinements.

Foundation — Whatever is touching the floor is considered the foundation of the yoga posture and should remain securely rooted when holding poses and when transitioning in and out of poses. The breath is thought to be part of the foundation because it supports this physical rooting and offers a great reminder to expand into whatever part of the body is touching the ground. This will protect a woman's joints, such as the wrists, from getting compressed.

General Form — The general form is the 'shape' and general structure that best supports good alignment in the posture. It also connects with the foundation when referring to the stance width and distance of the pose. Maintaining good general form allows the lines of energy to flow steadily, helping to circulate prana to all parts of the body and support proper muscle function. During pregnancy, the general form of certain poses will change to support joint laxity and balance as a woman's center of gravity changes. (i.e. For most women, stances in standing poses become shorter as the pregnancy progresses.) A woman should attempt to move towards the best general form she can without compromising the integrity of her muscles, ligaments and joints.

Primary Energy Flows — Refers to the pulsation between the integration and extension of the muscles and bones in the postures.

Integration — Engaging the muscles before stretching them helps to establish more stability and incorporates all the different parts of our body. The process of integration begins by first hugging the muscles onto the bones to create a sweet and sensitive engagement (as opposed to gripping, or hardening the muscles). The direction of the energy in the body moves from the skin, to the muscles, to the bones, resulting in an even tone on all sides of the body.

Once muscles are engaged, one can then engage the energy of the body into midline. For example, isometrically squeezing the legs towards each other is one way to create the engagement to the midline. Then, following both muscular engagement and an energetic focus toward the midline of the body, the energy of the body can be drawn from the periphery, such as fingertips and toes, into the core for support.

Extension — Once the muscles are engaged fully and the joints of the body are protected, lengthening out from the core fully without disengaging the muscles becomes more balanced. This pulsation of integration and extension requires focus, since most people, if they are not paying attention, will continually over stretch the same area of the muscle they are working. In pregnancy, relaxin is opening muscle tissue and joints. Therefore it is even more important that a pregnant woman maintain good muscle engagement as she stretches.

Refinements — After the breath, foundation, general form and primary energy flows are implemented, there are more refinements that offer maximal support for the postures. Here are some important tips to remember:

Top of the shin forward, base of the shin back — This helps to avoid hyperextension in the knees, which is very common in pregnancy and even postnatal. Engage the calves and press the mounds of the big toes forward to activate.

Thighs back first, then tailbone down — Root and widen the inner thighs, sitting bones and lower back before drawing in the tailbone and lengthening the lower back, to maintain integrity in the hip joint and lumbar spine.

Shins in, thighs out — This helps to track the knee joint and also supports opening the hips. The thighs must be integrated fully into the hip socket before widening.

Maintain length in sides of body — Allow the breath to support creating more space in the torso from hip to arm pit, allowing the armbones to float upward in line with the base of the neck.

Root the palate, armbones, and waistline back before extending — Sliding the palate, shoulders and waistline into the back of the body aligns the skeletal body more optimally, allowing for more stability and integrity before stretching.

Engage scapulas onto the back before expanding them — Particularly the bottom tips of the shoulder blades should be securely on the back before widening them. Make sure the breath is expanding into the ribcage before engaging scapulas.

PRENATAL YOGA

Prenatal yoga provides the foundation to support and empower a woman throughout all stages of her pregnancy. It builds confidence and trust — infusing a positive attitude that carries a woman through birth and into the threshold of motherhood.

Yoga increases overall strength and flexibility, helping to alleviate many common prenatal ailments such as low back pain, sciatica, fatigue, and nausea. Practicing regularly can help reduce swelling and inflammation around the joints, promoting circulation of blood and oxygen throughout the body. As the baby grows and there is less space for mom's internal organs, the fluid movements of yoga support both healthy digestion and regularity. Through optimally aligning the physical body, yoga opens the hips, supports the spine, and tones the pelvic floor muscles, better preparing a woman for both labor and physical birth.

Yoga also encourages a woman to trust in her greater connection to the Universe, providing the emotional support to let go of unwarranted (but completely normal) fears and step into the flow of Grace in the most natural and sublime way. Through connecting to the breath, a woman learns to deeply relax and tune in to the natural rhythms inside — reducing anxiety and stress. Yoga empowers a woman to feel deeply connected to her baby during pregnancy.

Group prenatal yoga classes provide a resourceful community of support and often lead to new friendships for mom (and baby). Sharing personal experiences and information can help to quiet anxious feelings and aid in decision-making. Being a part of a yoga studio also offers a perfect haven for a pregnant woman to connect to a larger community of open-hearted people.

Things to remember while practicing yoga:

- Keep the breath smooth and even — avoid any breathing exercises that hold the breath.
- Always create space for the baby — use props when necessary.
- Never push or force a pose — attune to the body, mind, and breath to know when to back off or come out of a pose completely.
- Keep feet at least hip width apart.
- Take as many breaks as needed.
- Strength over flexibility — keep back muscles strong.
- Engage the transverse abdominals, particulaly when transitioning in and out of poses.
- Maintain good postural alignment.
- Practice kegels regularly (see page 29).

- Keep water nearby, rest, take bathroom breaks when needed.
- Do not overheat! Excessive heat can raise body temperature and cause dehydration, potentially leading to fetal stress. American College of Obstetricians and Gynecologists (ACOG) recommend that pregnant women never let their core body temperature rise above 102.2° F.
- Do savasana on the left side with any necessary props to bring maximum blood flow and oxygen to the baby.
- Everyday is a new day. Check in and listen to how the body feels.

What to avoid in yoga practice:

- Jumping in or out of poses, including chaturanga dandasana.
- Low back twists and anything that closes the belly.
- Deep lunges, which can strain the ligaments in the front of the pelvis and destabilize the sacrum due to the hormone relaxin. Focus on strengthening muscles in the legs, gluteus and around the pelvic floor while stretching.
- Abdominal crunches that engage the rectus.
- Overstretching — particularly the belly and the ligaments around the pelvis and the sacrum. Go slowly into backbends and hip openers with increased engagement (once ligaments are overstretched, they can remain that way after pregnancy).
- Arm balances that 'crunch' the abdomen or create less space in the belly.
- Forward bends that compress the belly.
- Lying flat on the back after the 4th month — helps avoid the weight of the baby pressing into the inferior vena cava (vein to heart). This may result in dizziness in the mother and loss of blood and oxygen to mother and baby. To be safe, elevate the head and heart with a blanket at least five degrees.

Poses to be cautious of:

- Students new to yoga should not do inversions. Experienced practitioners should consider limiting inversions and avoiding any transitions that may be over jarring.
- Backbends can overstretch ligaments and abdominals and destabilize the sacrum.
- Pigeon — this deep hip opener can strain the groins and cause sacral shifts. It can be difficult for beginners to get into and hard on the knees. Experienced practitioners should make sure they are fully engaging and integrating the muscles of the body in this pose during pregnancy. Once they are overstretched, ligaments may not return to their pre-pregnancy state.
- Balancing poses that may create instability. Use the wall to avoid falling.

Modifying a non-prenatal yoga class:

The following modifications are useful if prenatal classes are not available, or if a pregnant woman wishes to continue taking open classes:

- A pregnant woman should inform the teacher of her pregnancy and any specific conditions/injuries that may be relevant.
- Have two blocks, a strap, a bolster, and/or extra blankets nearby.
- Modify all twists by 'opening up' in the opposite direction (rather than constricting the belly).
- When moving one leg forward from down dog to the top of the mat, bring the foot and leg out, up, and around from the side of the hip then back to the center of the mat (avoid crunching the belly).
- Keep the hands elevated on blocks for lunges and both hands inside the bent front leg.
- Bring the knees to the floor for chaturanga, and place a bolster or blanket under the thighs for cobra (to give the belly more space). Or skip both of these poses.
- Try to do Prenatal Sun Salutations instead of traditional Sun Salutations (see page 97):
    - Start at the back of the mat with a bolster or blocks in front.
    - Fold into uttanasana with hands on a bolster or blocks.
    - Walk hands from uttanasana to down dog.
    - Modify chaturanga with knees on the floor.
    - Do cobra with a bolster under thighs, or skip it and do extra push-ups or a seated shoulder stretch.
    - Walk hands back to feet from down dog to uttanasana.
- Use the wall when needed for all balancing poses, especially for inversions.
- Do not partner up with inexperienced students; a pregnant woman should consider partnering only with the teacher.
- Follow the "what to avoid" list on page 27 regardless of what everyone else is doing. Take malasana or virasana and practice kegels if the class is doing poses not suitable for a pregnant woman.
- Read the Prenatal Yoga Quick Reference Page (page 50) before practicing.
- Do savasana on the left side, using props to increase comfort.
- Don't forget to drink water!

KEGELS

Kegels are pelvic floor exercises originally developed by Dr. Arnold Kegel to help women with problems controlling urination. They are designed to strengthen, and give a woman voluntary control of, her pelvic floor muscles. The pelvic floor muscles are a group of muscles that attach to the front, back and sides of the bottom of the pelvis and sacrum. They are like a hammock or a sling, and they support the bladder, uterus, and rectum by wrapping around the urethra, vagina and rectum. A daily kegel practice will help to maintain and restore lost muscle tone due to pregnancy and childbirth. An easy way to locate the pelvic floor muscles is to stop and start the flow of urine while on the toilet, although this is not recommended to do as an exercise! Kegels may require a bit of concentration at first to build awareness on how to strengthen, and relax, the proper muscles. They can be done regularly throughout a woman's pregnancy, unless she is experiencing pelvic pain from hypertonic muscles, which requires professional attention and support. Many midwives and pelvic floor specialists recommend doing less kegels and more perineal massage after 36 weeks to relax the pelvic floor muscles and better prepare them for childbirth.

Kegel Exercises

• **Elevator lifts** — On your first cycle of breath, visualize all the deep muscles of the pelvic floor opening and relaxing. On your next inhalation, lift the deep hammock of muscles 'up' like they are a rising elevator. Start from the ground up, slowly isolating each floor until the 4th floor. Hold for four counts at the top floor (without holding the breath) and then release the muscles slowly, holding at each floor for a count until the ground floor. Then relax completely for a full cycle of breath. Repeat 3-4x, once or twice a day.

• **Slow Release Kegels** — Similar to the elevator lifts, begin your first cycle of breath relaxing all the muscles of the pelvic floor. On your next inhalation, slowly lift the muscles for the count of five, and slowly lower them down for the count of five, maintaining engagement on the way down, relaxing at the bottom. Repeat 10x, once or twice a day.

• **Quick Kegels** — tighten and relax muscles muscles continuously in pulses for 30 seconds to one minute. Try doing while holding a yoga posture.

Kegel exercises are also imperative to do AFTER the baby is delivered. Many women find their pelvic floor muscles so stretched that they have difficulty laughing hard or sneezing without the escape of some urine. Kegels will strengthen the inner pelvic muscles and may even make sexual intercourse more enjoyable. If there is any pelvic pain after birth, a woman should stop this exercise and see a pelvic floor specialist first.

SQUATTING

An essential part of prenatal and postnatal exercise is squatting. In conjunction with doing kegels, keeping your gluteus muscles strong supports overall pelvic floor health. Considered the birthing position in many cultures, squatting can increase the pelvic floor substantially and should be practiced regularly throughout pregnancy to aid in vaginal childbirth. If it is difficult for a woman to get her heels to the ground, she should place a blanket underneath them to stabilize the legs and help get extension in the spine. Squatting is a great place to practice kegels and can be done comfortably leaning against a wall and sitting on a block. In addition, longer squats (at least one minute) with the support of the wall can be great practice for the endurance of a contraction.

Once a woman reaches her third trimester, she should place a block or two underneath her sitting bones while squatting against the wall. This is to ensure that the muscles and ligaments in the pelvic floor do not overstretch due to the excess weight from the baby. Place the block in a horizontal position under the sitting bones, and use more than one block if needed.If the baby is breech, a woman should no longer squat after 34 weeks to avoid the baby's buttocks from getting lodged into her pelvis. If a woman has hemorrhoids (which are common during pregnancy) she should avoid squatting as soon as they develop.

MEDITATION AND IMAGERY

It is important for a woman to give herself quiet time everyday to reduce stress and create a deeper connection with herself and her baby. Meditation awakens this inner relationship and opens the heart to experience more joy and trust. Meditation can help a woman explore her deepest hopes and fears about pregnancy and being a parent, and support her in visualizing the birth she wants. It also can help her more easily express her feelings to others with love and trust. Regular practice increases positive emotions like love and compassion and helps to dissolve negative emotions and fears. It also strengthens the immune system, calms the nervous system, and increases brain function.

A wonderful way for a woman to honor the powerful time of pregnancy is to create a sacred place in her house (even just a spot) to spend time breathing, visualizing, and meditating daily. She can decorate the area with images that inspire and empower her, and take refuge in this sacred space during labor.

During pregnancy, I recommend sitting in virasana or sukhasana using blocks or blankets under the sitting bones. To begin the process of meditation, it may be helpful to use a timer. Start with ten minutes (or less) and then gradually increase the time as it becomes easier to sit longer. Try to use a timer with a soft chime rather than a jarring ring. Put on soothing music to help encourage a greater ability to 'let go.' Expand the breath evenly, allowing the mind to rest on its natural pulsation. Once the mind has been drawn inward and the body feels calm, allow the breath to soften. Let the whole body simply pulsate, visualizing each cell filled with healing energy and light. Continue to visualize the same for the baby, creating a deep feeling of connection and peace within. Guided meditation CDs provide another helpful resource for beginning a meditation practice. Some women even like to play them during early stages of labor to help relax. The following affirmations can be brought into meditation to help ease a woman's fears about childbirth:

- "I feel deeply connected to this miracle of life growing within me."
- "I trust that everything will be exactly the way it is meant to be."
- "I open and surrender to the Divine energy that is guiding the baby and me."
- "With every breath, I feel stronger yet more deeply relaxed."
- "My body knows what to do; I can relax."
- "As the uterus contracts, it's just an amazing 200 lbs of PRESSURE, not pain."
- "The Goddess and I dance together during contractions."

Meditating on the Goddess Within

The very power and source of the feminine energy in the Universe is within you. Listen to her in your heart; feel her deeply in each breath. As you develop your inner wisdom, trust your intuition. She is always available, providing you with infinite power and strength.

Envision the oldest image of the Goddess in your mind. Historically she is depicted as a large-bellied, robust woman, sculpted into figurines or drawn on cave walls. Her pregnant proportions represent the abundance that the Earth provides and the very source of our most fertile abilities as women to conceive and give birth.

As the mother Goddess, ruling completely the cycles of Nature, she is connected with both birth and death, and guarantees that death must occur with any new life. She is also the Cosmic Mother, overseeing the transitions of both life and death, to life again. On this cosmic level, she is the Goddess of Supreme Sound, Para Vac. In her most primordial form she is the entire cycle from silence through sound and back again – OM.

The cyclical nature of OM is expressed through the resonance of A–U–M and silence. The three sounds of A–U–M are accompanied by three stages of the creative cycle– creation, sustenance and dissolution, and are surrounded by a 4th aspect of Supreme silence, Turya. From silence, the sound of creation arises, and to silence sound returns.

Each syllable represents a different form of the Goddess and can be chanted as a celebration of our connection to Nature's most primordial essence of OM:
A – Kali – the original Mother, darkness, new beginnings & endings; absorptive energy
U – Saraswati – the emergence of expression, sound & light; creative energy
M – Lakshmi – celebrating the abundance of beauty & life; sustaining energy

MANTRA AND SOUND

The practice of vocalizing in prenatal yoga can be a great tool for a woman to release unwanted tension and tightness, free up her inhibitions and uplift her spirits. The baby too loves hearing the soothing vibrations of the mother's voice and often will become either excited or comforted by the rhythm of the vibration. Once a woman becomes comfortable with her 'sound,' she may find that she enjoys chanting mantra to herself and baby, both during and after birth.

Here are a few mantras a woman can do to practice vocal toning throughout her pregnancy. She may discover one mantra resonating more deeply than others and if so, spend more intimate time with that particular mantra. While focusing on the sound, she can allow herself to fully relax into its rhythm, as well as its supportive intention.

Bijas for Seven Chakras: (energy centers found along the midline of the body)

       LAM – Muladhara chakra (base of the spine)

       VAM – Swadhisthana chakra (lower abdomen)

       RAM – Manipura chakra (solar plexus)

       YAM – Anahata chakra (heart)

       HAM –Vishuddha chakra (throat)

OM – Ajna chakra (third eye)

Silence – Sahasrara chakra (crown of the head)

Kali/Shri mantra: place your two fingers on the energy centers while repeating bijas:

OM

AIM – third eye

HRIM – earth/muladhara

SHRIM – throat

AIM – third eye

KLIM – naval

SAU HA – heart

Bijas for Balance and Transformation:

SAA – Infinity, totality of the cosmos

TAA – Life (birth of form from infinity)

NAA – Death (or transformation)

MAA – Rebirth

This mantra describes the continous cycle of life and creation. It helps to balance the hemisheres of the brain, increase intuition and support us through times of transition, including pregnancy and birth.

Invocation to Lord Ganesha

OM GAM GANAPATAYE NAMAH

Om! Let us meditate on the benign face of Lord Ganesha, the face of Grace itself.

Gayatri Mantra: for Healing

Om bhur bhuva svaha

Tat savitur varenyam

Bhargo devasya dimahi

Dhiyo yo nah prachodayat

May there be peace on all planes.

I meditate on the most brilliant splendor of the divine sun.

May the energy of the sun stimulate our intellect,

And take right action at the right time.

EDUCATION

Research

Spending time researching pregnancy and birth, through online resources, books, and professionals, may be useful for a pregnant woman to understand what is going on within and empower her to trust the pregnancy and birthing process (see the Suggested Reading List on page 110).

Learning about the baby's stages of growth throughout the pregnancy will create a deeper connection between a woman and her baby. It also will help her better understand her own physical changes. Look online for pregnancy sites that offer daily or weekly updates (see the What's happening with Mama and Baby section on page 41).

Community

Networking through the yoga community can offer a woman lasting relationships that honor and empower her choices. Sharing experiences with other pregnant women provides support and a deeper understanding of possible prenatal and birth experiences. Exploring childbirth options, as well as vaccination and circumcision options, will allow a woman to feel more confident during critical decision-making.

Doula

Research the assistance of a doula to provide physical, emotional, and informational support for women and their partners during labor and birth. The word doula in Greek means 'one who serves a woman' and now has become known as a professional trained in childbirth. The doula's main role is to help women have safe and empowering birthing experiences. Research has shown using a doula decreases the overall cesarean rate, shortens labor, and reduces epidurals and the use of analgesia. Visit dona.org for more information on doulas and locating a doula in your area.

Labor Preparation

Learn common positions that support labor and practice regularly. Yoga postures like L-pose, all fours or modified child's pose on a bolster can all support low back pain in labor and keep baby in optimal fetal position during pregnancy.

PRENATAL NUTRITION

Eating well during pregnancy is essential for the health of both mother and baby. A nutritious and balanced diet will not only help a woman feel (and look) better throughout her pregnancy, it will lay the foundation for a lifetime of health for her child. The old saying, "you are what you eat" is never more fitting than during pregnancy — mom needs to remember that what she ingests goes directly to her baby. She should consider limiting or avoiding all foods and substances that could negatively affect the growing fetus — including caffeine, refined sugar, smoking, and alcohol. A prenatal vitamin recommended by a health practitioner or nutritionist will help to supplement certain crucial vitamins for baby's healthy development.

EATING WELL:
- Creates a more balanced physical and emotional state.
- Decreases the likelihood of morning sickness, fatigue, and constipation.
- Helps to expand blood volume to meet the increased demands pregnancy makes on the body. Blood bathes and washes over the placenta to help the exchange of oxygen and nutrients.
- Ensures that the uterus and other tissues grow and increase in elasticity and helps the baby grow to his or her full potential.
- May lower the risk of complications like infections, anemia, gestational diabetes, prematurity, pre-eclampsia, toxemia, low birth weight, stillbirth, brain damage, and mental retardation.
- Helps to produce good, healthy breast milk.
- Supports a faster recovery for the mother after birth.

Good nutrition for a pregnant woman begins with paying attention to food choices, and taking care to eat a variety of foods to ensure adequate nutrient intake. A pregnant woman should consult with her healthcare practitioner for the desirable amounts and proper intake of folic acid, iron, calcium, fluids, and protein. Pregnant women may also want to drink purified water instead of tap water to avoid lead, excess chlorine, metals, and synthetic hormones. Choosing organic foods whenever possible will reduce exposure to pesticides, insecticides, antibiotics, hormones, and other potentially harmful chemicals.

It is recommended for pregnant women to consume approximately 150 additional calories per day during the first trimester, and 300 additional calories per day during the second and third trimesters. Eating several small meals each day allows digestion to occur at a slower, steadier, and more balanced pace. This will help to stabilize blood sugar levels-- reducing nausea and heartburn. A pregnant mother needs to increase her consumption of protein, as well as fruits, nuts, green leafy vegetables, and grains. Fruits and vegetables provide critical vitamins and minerals, as well as fiber to aid digestion. In addition to increasing caloric intake while pregnant, nursing requires consumption of 400-700 more calories per day.

Protein is required for growth, maintenance, and repair of all cells, and is vital for nearly every process in the body, including metabolism, digestion, and transportation of nutrients and oxygen in the blood. It is also important for the production of antibodies, which fight infection and illness, and promote the health of hair, nails, skin, and bones. Protein is crucial for a baby's growth, especially during the second and third trimesters. Poultry, eggs, beans, and tofu are good sources of protein. Fish is an excellent source of protein and omega-3 fatty acids, which can promote baby's brain development. However, it is important to avoid fish that is potentially high in mercury.

Vitamin C, found in citrus fruits, strawberries, honeydew, papaya, broccoli, cauliflower, brussel sprouts, green peppers, tomatoes, and leafy greens, helps absorb iron, strengthens the immune system, and promotes healthy gums.

Vitamin A is found in dark green vegetables, carrots, pumpkins, sweet potatoes, spinach, water squash, turnip greens, beet greens, apricots, and cantaloupe. Approximately 770 mcg of vitamin A are recommended daily during pregnancy, most of which is obtained through a balanced diet. Take care not to exceed 3,000 mcg per day, as excess of vitamin A may be associated with fetal malformations.

Iron is found in beans, apricots, lentils, lean meat, eggs, seaweed, greens, barley, pumpkin seeds, oat bran, blackstrap molasses, dried fruit, and soy beans, and is crucial for blood cell formation. Iron also carries oxygen in muscles, and may lower susceptibility to stress and disease. The recommended intake of iron for a pregnant woman is 27 mg per day. It is best not to take calcium and iron supplements together, as they compete for absorption, whereas vitamin C is beneficial for iron absorption.

Calcium, found in dairy products, calcium-fortified soy milk, and dark green vegetables, helps build a baby's bones and teeth. Dairy products also have vitamin D and protein. Pregnant women require approximately 1,000 mg of calcium per day. One cup of milk contains approximately 245 mg of calcium, whereas one cup of enriched soy milk contains approximately 300 mg. Cheese has a concentrated amount of calcium, with one gram containing approximately the same amount as one cup of milk or yogurt. A growing baby requires a considerable amount of calcium for healthy development. If a pregnant woman lacks adequate calcium in her diet, her body will use its own calcium for the growth of her baby. This decreases bone mass and increases the risk of osteoporosis.

Folic Acid, found in dark leafy green vegetables, veal, and legumes, is important to help prevent neural tube complications such as spina bifida. A pregnant woman requires at least .4 mg of folic acid per day.

Whole grains like quinoa, brown rice, spelt, kamut, corn, millet, amaranth, and sprouted grains are rich in B vitamins, which help the body process stress, and can help with mood elevation.

Healthy fats are necessary for the body to stay in good health. Healthy fats, omega-3 and omega-6 fatty acids, must be supplied by diet, especially from plant foods and from fish that eat microscopic plants. Fatty acids are healthy for heart and brain functions. Sources include fish (especially salmon, shrimp, and sardines), walnuts, ground flaxseed, and flaxseed oil. Avocados are a good plant source of healthy fat and are also high in potassium, which is important for critical heart and cell functions. It is recommended that a pregnant woman consumes approximately 2,000 mg of potassium per day.

WHAT TO AVOID?

Certain substances are best avoided during pregnancy, including caffeine, alcohol, tobacco, drugs and certain prescription medications. Although fish is a great source of protein and omega-3 fatty acids, it should be consumed in moderation during pregnancy due to potentially high mercury content. Raw or undercooked fish, as well as shellfish, especially oysters and clams, should be avoided. Pregnant women may have a stronger reaction if exposed to foodbourne illness-inducing bacteria. It is recommended to limit fish consumption to 12 oz per week, and to avoid swordfish, king mackerel, tilefish, marlin and shark.

Caffeine is difficult for the baby to metabolize, and may be associated with low birth weight and miscarriage because of its potential to induce uterine contractions. It is best to limit caffeine consumption to 300 mg per day, or less. One 8 oz cup of coffee contains approximately 150 mg, whereas black tea contains approximately 80 mg. Chocolate and caffeinated soda also contain caffeine. It is best to limit consumption of these substances. As a diuretic, caffeine reduces the amount of fluid in a woman's body. It can also be attributed to preventing absorption of iron, a nutrient crucial to the baby's healthy growth and development.

Saturated fats and fats to avoid include margarine, cream, heavy salad dressing, vegetable oil, fried foods, partially hydrogenated and hydrogenated oils.

Sweeteners containing saccharin, aspartame, acesulfame-K, and sucralose are discouraged during pregnancy because they can cross the placenta and may remain in fetal tissues. High fructose corn syrup and corn syrup solids are also best avoided. Healthier alternatives include agave nectar, brown rice syrup, maple syrup, stevia, blackstrap molasses, and pasteurized honey.

Food cravings are completely normal during pregnancy, and experienced by almost two-thirds of pregnant women. It is okay to satisfy these cravings, as long as the food provides energy or an essential nutrient. However, if the craving interferes with a woman's consumption of other necessary nutrients, it is best that she practices moderation and balance in her diet.

THE THREE TRIMESTERS

FIRST TRIMESTER — (first 12 weeks)

For many women, the first trimester can be an exciting time — particularly if it's the first pregnancy. As the body begins its miraculous reshaping and hormonal levels change, it also can be a bumpy ride! Some women experience extreme nausea throughout the day, while others are fortunate to feel nothing, or just a little sick in the morning hours. Eating a few raw oats before getting up out of bed (and waiting 20 minutes for them to absorb the stomach acids) can sometimes alleviate this nausea. It is common for women to feel extra tired or hungry — both with good reason considering how much work the body is doing. There are always the lucky ones that feel perfectly fine throughout their entire pregnancy!

The following is a general list of some things to look for in the first trimester:

- Hormone levels increase.
- Mood swings and anxiety.
- Frequent urination (particularly at night as urination helps to eliminate fluid accumulating in the tissues during the day).
- Water retention.
- Feelings of nausea and fatigue.
- Increased appetite.
- Breast size may increase (preparing for breastfeeding).
- Joints between the pelvic bones widen and become more movable around the tenth or eleventh week. Separating bones can pinch the sciatic nerve.
- Constipation.
- Sensitivity to tastes and smells.

SECOND TRIMESTER — (13-26 weeks)

Usually by the second trimester the nausea subsides and energy levels go up (unfortunately not always). Women may find themselves seeking more physical activity and enjoying the company of others. All of the senses in the body heighten and certain smells or tastes are repulsive while others become extraordinary. The second trimester is generally thought of as the 'best' time in pregnancy, enabling travel or pursuing interests that may be difficult once the baby arrives.

- By the 5th month, a woman may be able to feel the movements of the fetus (although they actually begin much earlier around 7-8 weeks).
- Waist becomes thicker, womb swells.
- Weight gain.
- Blood volume increases.
- Blood pressure lowers.
- Line from navel to pubic region may darken.
- Increase in salivation.
- Increase in sweat production, which helps eliminate waste.
- Cramps in legs and feet.
- Varicose veins.
- Vivid dreams.
- General fears (baby disabilities, death, parenting concerns, etc.).

THIRD TRIMESTER — (27-38+ weeks)

By the third trimester, women are likely to slow down as the weight of the baby makes it more difficult to get around and breathe. Taking naps will help keep energy levels up. Eating smaller meals and more frequently will help alleviate heartburn due to lack of space in the stomach. Balance may become an issue and swelling in the feet, ankles, and hands are all common. Towards the end of the term, the uterus begins to prepare for its big push by contracting in what is known as 'false labor,' or Braxton Hicks contractions. Other symptoms in the third trimester include:

- Shortness of breath due to pressure on the lungs from the uterus.
- Diaphragm may be moved as much as an inch.
- Widening of the rib cage to allow for more breath.
- Stomach pushed up, indigestion.
- Difficulty sleeping.
- Walking differently for balance, leaning back to counter weight.
- Back aches (from leaning back), and pelvic joints more separated.
- Possible swelling (edema) in extremities (feet, ankles, hands).
- Uterus contracts and hardens (Braxton Hicks).
- Abdominal muscles separate.
- Fear and excitement about labor and delivery.
- A greater desire to 'nest.'

WHAT'S HAPPENING WITH MAMA & BABY?

FIRST TRIMESTER:
Month One (Weeks 1-4)
What's Happening with Mama?

A woman's first few months of pregnancy are the perfect time to reflect and make lifestyle changes in preparation for nourishing and welcoming a new life. It is not unusual for a woman to be unaware of her pregnancy during the first month, and common indications of pregnancy, including tiredness, nausea, tenderness of breasts, moodiness, and frequent urination, may be overlooked until the first menstrual period is missed. Don't stress if you did something 'not recommended' during this time, just begin to make healthy lifestyle changes as soon as you realize you are pregnant.

What's Happening with Baby?

Baby is a microscopic fertilized egg, which, after repeated cell division, becomes a ball of cells that will grow to become your baby's body. In this embryonic state, baby is nourished by a yolk sac, while all major organs begin to form. At the end of the first month, baby is about the size of a small pea, and weighs less than an ounce!

What to do?

Beginning in the first month, it is important to stay healthy by drinking plenty of water, eating fresh organically grown foods, getting sufficient rest, and steering clear of viral illness. Eliminating depleting elements such as smoking, alcohol, drugs, as well as certain over-the-counter medications (check with your healthcare provider) will help to create an optimal environment for your new baby. As far as yoga goes, you can continue your regular practice if it feels okay—keeping in mind not to overdo it.

Month Two (weeks 5-8)
What's Happening with Mama?

You might 'feel' more pregnant, as estrogen and progesterone levels increase substantially. These hormone shifts may lead to mood swings, as well as swelling of the breasts due to increased milk ducts. You may experience nausea and fatigue this month, which will greatly diminish by the end of the first trimester. By the end of this month, your uterus will have expanded to roughly the size of a tennis ball.

What's Happening with Baby?

Beginning with the central nervous system, baby's body systems are starting to form. Baby's face, eyes, ears, and mouth are forming, and brain cells are growing. By six weeks, baby is surrounded by amniotic fluid, creating a controlled and protected environment.

The baby begins to move around seven or eight weeks, stretching his or her arms and legs. By the end of this month, the placenta takes over and the baby is officially called a fetus— approximately an inch in length and less than an ounce in weight.

What to do?

This is a crucial time to continue healthy diet and lifestyle choices. Stay up on your vitamins as recommended by your healthcare practitioner, and limit caffeine intake. You can reduce acid indigestion by limiting certain elements such as caffeine, milk, citrus, and carbonation. Baby is susceptible to birth defects from now until the twelfth week, so take extra care to provide good nutrients for him or her. As you feel changes in your body, it's time to begin to modify your yoga. Don't over work (your heart rate should not go past 150 bpm), and remember to stay hydrated! Avoid excessive twisting as a precaution. If you feel sick, listen to your body and rest.

Month Three (weeks 9-12)

What's Happening with Mama?

Your body is adjusting to pregnancy, and will feel less tired as your heart acclimates to pumping an increased volume of blood to accommodate your baby. By the end of this month, risk of miscarriage and birth defects will be greatly reduced, as the critical period of early organ development will have passed. Your uterus is about the size of a grapefruit, and your clothing might begin to feel tight.

What's Happening with Baby?

Baby's nose, eyelids, eyebrows, eyelashes, nails, and skin are formed, and the soft skeletal cartilage has begun to turn into bone. By the end of this month, baby's body is covered by a downy hair called lanugo, and external genital organs are recognizable. Baby's heartbeat is growing stronger, and baby can roll over, open and close his or her mouth, swallow, make a fist, smile, and squint. Baby weighs approximately one ounce and is the size of a walnut.

What to do?

Continue your diet of whole grains, healthy fats, and nutrient-rich foods. Rest when you need to rest. As tiredness subsides nearing the end of the third month, stay active to avoid gaining excess weight. An ultrasound to determine baby's age, as well as other tests to screen for possible birth defects, are often done around this time.

Teacher tip:

Consider advising your students to lay low on jarring and jumping movements as a precaution to make sure everything sticks. While inversions done briefly are not necessarily problematic, the transitions up or down may not be ideal during this time.

SECOND TRIMESTER
Month Four (weeks 13-16)
What's Happening with Mama?

Entering your second trimester will likely bring a sense of relief and new calmness. As nausea subsides, your appetite will increase, and perhaps be accompanied by certain food cravings. Frequent urination is likely, especially during the night. Skin pigmentation on your face, breasts, arms, and nipples may change, and your waistline will likely begin to disappear as muscles and ligaments relax. As your body becomes accustomed to pregnancy, you may notice you have more energy. If you are choosing to practice inversions in yoga, keep the duration short and take care to land softly. Keep your knees on the floor in chaturanga and avoid putting weight directly on your belly.

What's Happening with Baby?

Baby is about 2 or 3 inches long and weighs around five ounces. The head is larger in proportion to the rest of the body, and gender is not yet fully decipherable. Baby's ears and eyes are mostly developed at this time. You may start to feel a slight fluttering sensation in your lower abdomen (called quickening). Recording this date as baby's first perceptible movement will help to determine when your baby is due.

What to do?

Improve your circulation by sleeping and resting on your left side. Stay hydrated, continue eating fresh organic foods as much as possible, and take care not to exceed recommended daily allowance for vitamin A. Stay active with walking and stretching!

Teacher Tip:

At the end of the fourth month, place a blanket under your student's head and upper back, at a five degree incline, to keep her head above her heart in savasana or when she is on her back. This will prevent the weight of the baby and growing uterus from pressing down on the vena cava (a major vein), which could result in cutting off oxygen supply and potentially cause fainting.

Month Five (weeks 17-20)
What's Happening with Mama?

As the risk of miscarriage has most likely passed, you may now comfortably share the good news of your pregnancy with the world. Your appetite will continue to increase, and the need for frequent urination may subside as your body adapts to pregnancy. Changes in skin pigmentation will continue, and your breasts may begin to produce colostrum. Nasal congestion, gum bleeding, and increased vaginal discharge are common during this month of pregnancy.

What's Happening with Baby?

Baby's body size is now catching up with its head, measuring approximately 4 inches in length. If baby's movements have not yet been perceptible, they will become so during this month. Baby's fingers and toes are defined, and heartbeat continues to become stronger. The downy hair, called lanugo, which covered baby at the end of month 3, will begin to grow more rapidly. This hair protects the baby, and will mostly disappear by the time of birth.

What to do?

Continue eating locally grown, unprocessed fresh foods whenever possible. Try eliminating caffeine entirely from your diet. Increase your intake of high-density lipoproteins- good cholesterol. Pamper yourself and your baby!

Month Six (weeks 21-24)

What's Happening with Mama?

You are now visibly pregnant. There may be some achiness in the lower abdomen, and sharp twinges on the sides of the belly, as ligaments supporting the uterus expand. There may also be pain in the ribcage or shortage of breath as baby begins to press upwards. It is common to feel overheated and appear flushed in the face as blood supply increases. Your heart and lungs are working much harder than normal! Sexual pleasure may return or increase during the sixth month.

What's Happening with Baby?

Baby is approximately 8-10 inches long, weighs about one pound, and is becoming very active, now able to turn over, suck his or her thumb, hiccup, and sleep. If a girl, baby's ovaries are formed and contain her lifetime supply of eggs. Baby has white eyelashes, and hair is beginning to grow on his or her head. Baby is covered with vernix, a white, creamy substance that protects the skin before birth.

What to do?

As baby grows, and more weight is carried by your body, continuing to pay attention to good alignment will help to keep you comfortable and protect your joints. Rest with your feet up, and take steps to reduce leg and foot cramps, informing your healthcare provider of any severe leg pain, tenderness, or swelling.

THIRD TRIMESTER
Month 7 (weeks 25-28)
What's Happening with Mama?

This is a nice month for mama! You will likely feel good, have a hearty appetite, and experience less mood swings. Your belly will be more pronounced, and you may notice stretch marks on your navel or thighs. As baby grows, he or she will begin to press on your stomach and diaphragm, causing possible indigestion and shortness of breath. Your pelvic joints will loosen in preparation for delivery, which may cause sciatic or back pain. Breast tenderness and leg cramps are also common during this month.

What's Happening with Baby?

Baby is still coated with vernix caseosa, and now has thin, translucent skin. He or she is around 13-16 inches long, weighs between 2 and 3 pounds, and is beginning to build up body fat, which will help to maintain a consistent body temperature upon delivery. Baby is beginning to practice breathing movements, can sense light changes, and can now hear the outside world over the sound of your heartbeat. If born prematurely, baby has a strong chance of survival.

What to do?

Allow yourself plenty of rest and breaks during the day, especially if you are feeling short of breath. Enjoy doing things to help calm your mind and connect to your baby, such as restorative poses and meditation. Continue to stay active and incorporate exercise into your daily routine, modifying yoga poses with props, and avoiding anything that closes the front of the body or overstretches your ligaments. Do your kegel exercises daily! Including yogurt with probiotics in your diet will help to reduce the risk of yeast infections, and calcium rich foods will help to reduce leg cramping.

Teacher Tip: In the third trimester, use support in squatting positions, such as malasana. This will help to prevent hemorrhoids and varicose veins.

Month 8 (weeks 29-32)
What's Happening with Mama?

If you've not already experienced shortness of breath and indigestion, you likely will begin to this month. Baby's growth will also likely cause more frequent urination and difficulty finding a comfortable sleeping position. You may experience painless contractions, called Braxton Hicks, which are your uterus's way of practicing for labor.

What's Happening with Baby?

Baby weighs around 4-6 pounds, and is 16-18 inches long. Baby is continuing to build a layer of fat, and his or her liver is storing iron in preparation for life outside the womb. Baby's kicks are strong and frequent. His or her regulating functions, including lungs, digestive system, and body temperature, still need to mature. In preparation for descent in birth, baby will usually turn head-down this month.

What to do?

Continue your vitamin-rich diet of organic whole grains, fruit, vegetables, adequate protein, and plenty of water. Soothe itchy skin with organic jojoba oil. Enjoy preparing your home to create a welcoming environment for your new family member.

Month 9 (weeks 33-36+)

What's Happening with Mama?

You are feeling ready for pregnancy to be over and looking forward to your baby's due date! You will likely experience Braxton Hicks contractions, if you haven't already done so. Swelling of ankles and lower back aches are common at this time, and your breasts will increase their production of colostrum. You may experience fluctuations of energy, alternating between fatigue and extra alertness. By the end of a pregnancy, the fluids in the body (cells, tissues, and blood) can increase up to 12 pints. The heart's pumping power also has to increase to meet the demands of the blood volume increase (9 pints).

What's Happening with Baby?

Baby is approximately 18 inches long, and weighs around 5-7 pounds. His or her heart and lungs are almost ready for life outside the womb, and senses of hearing and vision are developed. The lanugo (downy hair) covering baby has disappeared, and the creamy protective covering of vernix is diminishing. Baby is receiving mama's antibodies, as preparation for post-womb life. He or she will likely become less active as birth nears, and will tend to roll, rather than kick in the womb. Baby will descend in your pelvis approximately two weeks before birth, which will ease the pressure on your diaphragm and stomach, but increase the pressure on your bladder. The bones in baby's head are soft and flexible to allow more ease in delivery.

What to do?

Relax as much as possible! Continue to connect to your baby through breath, meditation, and restorative yoga poses. Enjoy long walks and taking time to prepare for your new child. Listen to your body-- rest when tired and take advantage of periods of higher energy, being careful not to overdo it.

PREGNANCY CONDITIONS

Here are some common pregnancy conditions and possible ways to alleviate discomfort.

Backaches — Maintain good posture. Try pelvic rocking, thigh stretches, prenatal massage, and visiting a chiropractor specializing in pregnancy.

Breech (at 30-35 weeks) — Put gentle pressure on baby's head to move. See spinningbabies.com. Try acupuncture, moxibustion (a traditional Chinese medicine technique that involves the burning of mugwort), and light or music between the legs. Try communicating with the baby.

Some yoga poses to support flipping the baby include:
* Quarter dog: knees on the floor, hips higher than the head and heart.
* Supported down dog with a block under the head or someone holding a strap around the hips and through the inner thighs.
* Supported backbends with a bolster, blanket, or blocks.
* Inverted L-pose (if comfortable).
* Headstand (if comfortable).

Carpal tunnel syndrome — Strengthen the wrists by engaging in good shoulder and upper back alignment. Elevate the heels of the hands on a blanket roll/towel during practice. Wearing a splint on the wrist at night also may help alleviate night pain.

Colds — Nettie pot the sinuses with un-iodized salt. Breathe in steam of chamomile tea. Take buffered vitamin C, zinc, and vitamin B. Consider homeopathic remedies.

Constipation — Eat plenty of fruits and vegetables. Increase water intake and other fluids, including prune juice.

Dehydration — Drink plenty of water. Stay out of the sun. Minimize caffeine.

Dizziness — Sit or lie down to avoid falling. When practicing yoga, do not bring arms over head, come into child's pose, and rest. Try Bach Flower Rescue Remedy.

Edema (swelling) — Drink plenty of water. Elevate legs up the wall if swelling is in the feet, ankles, or legs (lift the head above heart after the 4th month). Sleep on the left side. Avoid sitting or standing too long. If sudden or extreme swelling occurs, check with a health care professional to make sure it is not a sign of preeclampsia.

Excessive heat — Rest. Practice *sitali* breathing (cooling breath by sipping air through the tongue — see page 23). Stay well hydrated.

Headache — Due to dehydration: drink water, take electrolytes, and rest. From hormones: drink water, rest, massage lavender oil on temples (or peppermint oil after 16 weeks).

Heartburn — Eat smaller, more frequent meals. Remain upright for an hour after eating. Lying down can irritate the problem. Avoid spicy or greasy foods. Consider homeopathic remedies. Practice virasana/supta virasana with props as necessary.

Hemorrhoids — Practice legs up the wall (elevate the head and heart after the 4th month). Avoid squatting. Eat more fruits and vegetables, and drink more fluids.

Indigestion — Practice virasana/supported supta virasana. Drink mint tea. Avoid greasy and spicy foods. Eat smaller meals.

Insomnia — Drink chamomile tea. Avoid eating close to bedtime. Massage head and neck. Try calcium or magnesium supplements. Practice pelvic rocking. Massage lavender essential oil on feet. Go for a walk, meditate, and do yoga during the day.

Leg cramps — Flex and point foot to engage calf muscles (if they cramp while sleeping). Get adequate calcium intake. Dissolve four tablets of Magnesia Phosphorica 6X in a small glass of warm water. Practice seated (wide legged) forward bends like upavista konasana.

Nausea — Take some form of ginger, either candy or tea. Acupressure: press center point right below the wrist. Eat: have raw oats next to the bed and eat before sitting up. Make sure to have snacks handy when going out. Avoid inversions and backbends. Try standing thigh stretches.

Overdue (or due) — Massage pressure points: three fingers above inner ankle bone and hand at break between thumb and index finger. Exercise — walking or climbing stairs.

Pelvic pain — Regular exercise will help. Rest if painful, or try warm compresses. Try tightening a yoga strap around pubis and base of sacrum for support.

Placenta previa — (When the placenta grows in the lowest part of the uterus and covers all or part of the opening to the cervix.) Reduce activities, stay on bedrest, and see a doctor.

Preeclampsia (pregnancy hypertension) — To prevent elevated blood pressure, make sure to eat a well-balanced diet and rest. See a nutritionist specializing in prenatal care.

Restless leg syndrome — (Central nervous system disorder which causes an urge to move the legs, associated with an uncomfortable or unpleasant sensation.) Exercise/yoga to stretch and move area. Massage or wrap legs. Place pillow between legs at night. Increase iron intake.

Sciatica — Practice tadasana with a block between the legs. Practice standing thigh stretches and supta padangustasana.

Stretch marks — Eat the proper diet to promote healthy skin. Drink plenty of fluids. Keep the skin hydrated, and massage the belly with shea butter, vitamin E, or jojoba oil.

Supine hypotensive syndrome — Avoid lying flat on the back after the 4th month to prevent possible dizziness and drop of blood pressure caused by weight of uterus, baby, placenta, and amniotic fluids compressing the inferior vena cava, which may also reduce blood to mother's heart and amount of oxygen to baby.

Swelling — Practice virasana, legs up the wall (elevate the head and heart after the 4th month), and wrist and ankle circles. Stay well-hydrated.

Toxemia — (Elevated blood pressure, protein in urine, fluid retention, preeclampsia or eclampsia/maternal seizures.) This is a very serious condition that needs medical attention right away.

Varicose veins — Practice legs up the wall (use incline under back after the 4th month), exercise the pelvic floor and inner thigh muscles, use theraband for resistance with leg lifts, virasana. Avoid crossing your legs while sitting. Wear support pantyhose.

PRENATAL YOGA QUICK REFERENCE PAGE

Here are some general prenatal yoga tips and guidelines for all yoginis who have begun the amazing journey into motherhood. The first thing to remember is that every pregnancy is different, even for the same woman. It is always best to listen to your body and do only what feels right for you each day. If you are new to yoga, now is not the time to overdo it. Modify accordingly, especially when trying new poses. Concentrate on maintaining good alignment and breathing deeply.

1st trimester - the first four weeks: Don't stress if you did something 'not recommended.' Most women don't even know they're pregnant until at least the 5th week! As far as yoga goes, you can continue practicing if it feels okay, keeping in mind not to strain or overheat.

5-8 weeks: Now that you know you are pregnant, you'll start feeling the changes in your body. It's time to begin to modify your yoga. Don't over work and get dehydrated! (Your heart rate should not go past 150 bpm.) Avoid excessive twisting and abdominal 'crunches' as a precaution.

If you feel sick, listen to your body and rest more. Eat. Let go of the idea that you should have to have the perfect body when you're pregnant. It is fine to continue your regular yoga practice (being mindful of the precautions listed on pages 26-27 and paying close attention to how you are feeling), but it is also good to start learning how to modify your poses.

9-12 weeks: This is a nice time to back up your yoga practice even more and make sure everything sticks (risks of miscarriage and birth defects will drop substantially by the end of the month). Consider limiting inversions for this period, and avoiding any transitions that may be jarring. Refrain from deep lower belly twists. Take care in backbends not to overstretch the belly. You may have to ease up on these until they feel better and engage your transverse abdominals for more support. If you haven't been to a prenatal yoga class yet, now would be a great time to start.

2nd trimester: If you weren't feeling so great during your first trimester, rejoice, relief is in sight. The nausea should subside, and you may notice that you have more energy now. If you love inversions, now is the safest time to put them back in. Headstands and handstands can be done for short periods if they feel okay. Make sure to use a wall, or ask the teacher for support, because your center of gravity and ability to balance may shift from day-to-day. If inversions are new for you, wait until after your baby arrives to start. Your yoga practice should consist mainly of standing poses, squats, shoulder and hip openers, leg strengtheners and stretches, breathing exercises, transverse abdominal exercises and kegels. Keep your knees on the floor in chaturanga and do not do anything directly on your belly — your baby likes lots of space. Remember to continue to drink plenty of water.

By the end of the fourth month, because of your growing baby and uterus, lying flat on your back could put excessive weight on the vena cava (a major vein), which may cut off blood flow and oxygen to you and your baby. You will feel dizzy before the baby is in any danger. This does not happen for everyone, but to be safe, place a blanket under your head and upper back at a five degree incline to keep your head above your heart. The most optimal resting position is on your left side since this brings maximum blood flow to baby. Therefore, practice savasana on your left side.

3rd trimester: You're getting pretty good at knowing what you can and can't do by now. Continue to modify poses using props, and avoid doing anything that closes the front of your body and overstretches your ligaments. Keep your legs wide apart for seated poses, and don't push too far. Some days you'll have energy for your practice and other days you won't. Remember to do your kegel exercises regardless. Try doing more restorative poses to calm the mind and help you connect to your baby. This is such a magical time. Make sure you slow down enough to enjoy this miracle of life within you. If you haven't been to prenatal classes yet, now is the time. It's a wonderful way to connect with other women and make lasting new friendships for you and your baby.

ESSENTIAL OILS FOR PREGNANCY

Aromatherapy uses pure essential plant oils to enhance and restore health by stimulating the body's own natural healing process. There are different qualities or 'grades' of essential oils. It is very important for pregnant women to use the highest quality 'therapeutic' grade oils. This section includes a list of essential oils to avoid and a list of those that are safe for pregnant women to use during specific times of pregnancy and childbirth. I have noted whether they are 'safe throughout' (s.t.), or to be used only after a certain number of weeks. Essential oils should always be diluted in carrier oils during pregnancy. For topical treatments and massage, dilute two drops of essential oil for every one teaspoon of carrier oil. Carrier oils include vegetable oils, sweet almond oil, grape seed oil, jojoba oil, etc.

The following two companies have superb integrity and high quality therapeutic grade oils:

- Oshadhi: oshadhiusa.com
- Swiss Aromatics: originalswissaromatics.com

To introduce the use of essential oils during pregnancy, a woman may choose an appealing scent and place one drop on a tissue to inhale. If the smell is pleasant, she can then place the tissue inside her bra and enjoy it for the rest of the day. Other options include: adding essential oils to a bath (dilute three to seven drops mixed with a carrier oil before putting into bath), using a device to diffuse oils into a room (ceramic burner, electric diffuser, or vaporizer), and adding four drops to lukewarm water to soak feet, etc. I recommend that pregnant women try lavender oil, which has many wonderful therapeutic qualities and is safe to use throughout pregnancy.

It is best to avoid essential oils that are known to thin the blood or cause cramping or contractions. In general, a pregnant woman should err on the side of caution, particularly during the first trimester and consult with her doctor, midwife, or a practitioner trained in the application of essential oils during pregnancy. As it is obviously highly unethical to test on pregnant women, the following list of essential oils is based on knowledge of the general properties of each oil.

ESSENTIAL OILS TO AVOID DURING PREGNANCY

Basil   Lemongrass
Camphor   Myrrh
Cedarwood   Parsley
Cinnamon   Pennyroyal
Clove   Sage
Fennel   Sweet marjoram
Hyssop   Tansy
Juniper   Thyme

ESSENTIAL OILS TO BE USED WITH CAUTION DURING PREGNANCY

Chamomile, Roman (safe after 16 weeks)
Clary Sage (only late pregnancy)
Cypress (safe after 16 weeks)
Geranium (safe after 16 weeks)
Jasmine (safe after 16 weeks)
Peppermint (safe after 16 weeks)
Rose (safe after 16 weeks)
Rosemary (late pregnancy only, avoid if high blood pressure)

ESSENTIAL OILS SAFE TO USE DURING PREGNANCY

Bergamot   Orange
Frankincense   Patchouli
Grapefruit   Rosewood
Lavender   Sandalwood
Lemon   Tangerine
Mandarin   Tea Tree
Neroli   Ylang Ylang

Note — bergamot, lemon, mandarin, and orange essential oils are phototoxic (can cause skin irritation) and should not be used while in direct sunlight.

COMMON PREGNANCY CONDITIONS SUPPORTED BY ESSENTIAL OILS

It is important for a pregnant woman to seek the counsel of a qualified aromatherapist before administering essential oils on her own to alleviate ailments.

Backache: roman chamomile (after 16 wks), rosemary (late pregnancy), lavender (s.t.).

Depression and anxiety: bergamot (s.t.), roman chamomile (after 16 wks), frankincense (s.t.), geranium (after 16 wks), neroli (s.t.), ylang-ylang (s.t.), rose (after 16 wks).

Edema (swelling): geranium (after 16 wks), grapefruit (s.t.).

Lethargy: orange (s.t.), peppermint (after 16 wks).

Headaches: lavender (s.t.), peppermint (after 16 wks).

Healing damaged tissue: tea tree (s.t.), lavender (s.t.).

Hormonal balance: geranium (after 16 wks), jasmine (good for after childbirth), rose (good for after childbirth).

Indigestion: lavender (s.t.).

Immune system booster: lemon (s.t.), lavender (s.t.).

Induce labor/strengthen contractions: clary sage (only late pregnancy- stimulates and tones uterus).

Inflamed skin: lavender (s.t.).

Insomnia: lavender (s.t.).

Muscle spasm: roman chamomile (after 16 wks).

Nausea: lavender (s.t.), peppermint (after 16 wks).

Poor circulation: geranium (after 16 wks), lemon (s.t.).

Postpartum depression: vetiver, lemon, cedarwood, sandlewood, St. John's wort.

Relaxing, calming, optimism: jasmine (after 16 wks), roman chamomile (after 16 wks), mandarin (s.t.), rose (after 16 wks), sandalwood (s.t.).

Settles digestive tract: mandarin (s.t.), orange (s.t.), peppermint (after 16 wks), lavender (s.t.).

Settles nervous system: mandarin (s.t.), neroli (s.t.), rose (after 16 wks).

Stress: lavender (s.t.), frankincense (s.t.), geranium (after 16 wks).

Stretch marks: neroli (s.t.).

Varicose veins/hemorrhoids: cypress (after 16 weeks).

PERINEAL MASSAGE USING CARRIER OIL

During the last six weeks of a woman's pregnancy, she may want to try massaging her perineum for five or six minutes a day to prevent tearing or the need for an episiotomy during delivery.

To begin, she can take a warm bath or shower to help relax the tissues. Using a nut-based carrier oil such as almond oil, she can begin by simply massaging her perineum and lower vaginal wall. After a couple of minutes, she should begin to use both of her thumbs inside the vagina and press down towards her rectum. Maintaining steady pressure, she should move her thumbs in a "U" type movement, hold for 30-60 seconds, then release. If she feels a slight burning or tingling sensation, she can try relaxing her pelvic floor muscles. This is what she must do when the baby's head begins to crown in birth. At first this tissue will feel tight, but with time it will stretch and relax. The exercise should not be painful. She can seek her care provider's help if she has difficulty or questions.

PREPARING FOR LABOR AND BIRTH WITH YOGA

The extraordinary journey of pregnancy culminates in the process of giving birth. It is likely to be among the most powerful and monumental experiences for both the mother and child. Yoga supports this sacred passage by preparing a woman both physically and emotionally, while offering her resources for before, during labor, and even after the baby arrives.

During the last six weeks or so of pregnancy, a woman will experience many different sensations as her body innately prepares for birth. On a physical level, the ligaments in her pelvis are moving towards maximum softness to allow her pelvic and sacroiliac joints to expand. The uterus will begin contracting (Braxton Hicks), which may feel like a powerful tightening or hardening of the abdomen. Usually the baby's head begins to descend into the pelvis during the last four weeks (lightening), potentially increasing contractions. Once she notices a 'dropping' of the baby, she may feel less pressure on her diaphragm making it easier to breathe — but possibly more pressure on her bladder resulting in more frequent urination. (Note: 'lightening' prior to labor is more obvious with first time births because the uterine muscles are tighter and babies are under more downward pressure.)

By utilizing the breath, mantra (affirmations), specific yoga postures, and meditation, a woman can often alleviate discomfort in her lower back and pelvis. She can even maximize space in the birth canal for Optimal Fetal Positioning and baby's entrance into the world. These practices also help release stiffness and tension in her muscles, keeping her body softer and more capable of relaxing when needed. It is essential for a woman's pelvic floor to relax during childbirth to avoid unwanted tears or an episiotomy (a surgical incision through the perineum made to enlarge the vagina and assist childbirth).

BREATHING EXERCISES FOR LABOR

It is best for a woman to practice awareness of the breath throughout her pregnancy (see grounding breath on page 23). When she begins the first stage of labor she can return to the connection and familiarity of the breath to move her through her contractions. As the contractions build in strength, she should focus on her exhalation, relax as much as possible, and naturally let the inhalation begin. Repeat this cycle through the wave of each contraction until it ebbs.

There is no 'right' way to breathe. It is more important that a woman is comfortable with what she is doing, especially as the labor progresses into the second stage (bearing down). Some women are taught to take a huge breath, hold it, and push, while others may be encouraged to relax into the contraction and surrender. It is safe to encourage a woman to keep breathing deeply (this supplies maximum oxygen for herself and her baby), concentrate on opening and relaxing on her exhale, and center her awareness on releasing all tension in her pelvic floor to aid in the arrival of her baby. Relaxing the mouth and jaw is one way to help accomplish this.

MANTRAS (AFFIRMATIONS) FOR LABOR

Sound plays an important role in enabling a woman to let go. As the labor progresses, she will find it very difficult to tolerate outside sounds or disturbances. A woman may turn inward, finding a comfortable place to open to her deep primal urge to sound. Having a 'mantra,' which is simply a sound, syllable, or group of words that she can repeat over and over again, will help her move more deeply into a trance-like state. It also helps her relax her lips and mouth, which may have a similar effect on loosening her cervix.

Some possible mantras she can repeat are:
- 'Oooooommmmmmm.'
- 'Aaaaaaah, Uuuuuu, Mmmm' (Aum translates to Om).
- 'So hum' (I am that).

Some possible affirmations she can repeat are:
- 'Opening and surrendering.'
- 'Inhale/exhale.'
- 'Each contraction brings me closer to meeting my baby.'
- 'Wow, 200 lbs of pressure, not pain.'
- 'All is well.'
- 'With grace and ease.'
- 'I am (fill in the blank)' – i.e strong, ready, etc.
- 'Oh yes.'

OPTIMAL FETAL POSITIONING

Optimal Fetal Positioning can assist the baby in moving into, and maintaining, the best position from which to enter the world. This theory, developed by Jean Sutton, a midwife practicing in New Zealand, states that a woman's posture and movement during the final weeks of pregnancy can directly influence the baby's position in the womb. The ideal position for the baby is with his or her face facing the mother's back (Occiput Anterior position). At the end of pregnancy, if a woman can spend more time upright or on all fours, rather than leaning back in an armchair or couch, she has a better chance of allowing gravity to aid in naturally sliding the baby's head and spine (the heaviest parts of his or her body) into an Occiput Anterior (OA) position. From this optimal position, the baby has space to flex his or her chin to chest, and the smallest diameter of the baby's head leads the way through the birth canal.

Conversely, when the baby's back is toward the mother's back and his or her face is toward the mother's belly (Occiput Posterior position), this is known to result in longer ('back') labor. Opposite of the space provided in optimal positioning, this position limits the baby's ability to move his or her chin to chest and a larger diameter of the baby's head is entering the birth canal first.

Yoga postures that may help with Optimal Fetal Positioning:
- All fours
- Cat/cow
- L-pose at the wall
- Quarter dog
- Downward facing dog
- Prasarita padottanasana
- Upavista konasana
- Supported child's pose

YOGA POSTURES FOR LABOR

A woman will naturally move in a variety of positions during labor to help alleviate discomfort and relax her body. It is helpful for her to get to know the following yoga postures beforehand so she can support these natural instincts during labor.

Standing Tadasana: works with gravity to assist the baby moving downward and helps thin the cervix.

Modified Tadasana: leaning forward with her arms around a partner's neck, she can 'hang' on her exhalation and have her partner massage her back.

Supported Tadasana: put a strap around the top of a door and holding the strap with both hands, let her body 'hang' on her exhalations during contractions.

Supported Balasana (child's pose): knees wide, torso resting over a chair or pillows. This is a good position to have a partner massage her back.

Squatting: helps put pressure on the cervix to open and shortens the distance of the birth canal. This position is best to use as labor progresses as it makes contractions more intense.

Modified squatting: sitting on the edge of a chair with her knees wide, leaning forward.

Partner squatting: have a partner stand behind with his/her forearms under her armpits, allowing her to bend her knees half way and let go on contractions.

Supported deep squat: have a partner support her from behind in a squat or low chair.

All fours/pelvic rocking: relieves lower back pain by taking the weight of baby away from her spine. Also allows for less pressure on her tailbone.

Supported all fours: using the support of a chair or pillow for elbows, resting her weight forward.

Supported Savasana (on left side): good position for resting or sleeping, this helps her perineum relax to prevent tearing. This is the preferred position as opposed to lying on her back, which may slow down labor.

THE HORMONAL CONNECTION

Through yoga and meditation, a woman also learns to surrender more and more into her deeper states of consciousness, tapping into her most instinctive and primal self. This expansion of awareness, which is natural to feel at the end of pregnancy, will support her immensely if she can flow with it. It will also give her more ease and assurance that she is ready, regardless of how her labor progresses. As a woman invokes an overall sense of 'calm,' through conscious breathing, sound and movement, she stimulates the part of her autonomic nervous system known as the parasympathetic nervous system. This not only helps to lower her heart rate, blood pressure and energy consumption, but also to release the birthing hormones that aid her tremendously in labor and birth.

While it is completely normal to feel anticipation and anxiety surrounding the unknowns of labor, if a woman is highly stressed in early labor, she is stimulating the sympathetic nervous system, which has the opposite effect on the hormonal physiology of childbirth. Fear causes tension and tension causes pain. Excessive fear, feeling unsafe, or being disturbed during labor, shifts the blood supply to a woman's muscles and her heart, reducing blood supply to her uterus and baby. This 'fight or flight' response prolongs labor and can also have adverse effects on the baby's fetal heart rate pattern.

The more a woman can face her concerns and fears during pregnancy and open up to the intensity of labor, the more her body's natural wisdom can take over and help her give birth the way Mother Nature intended it to be. Yoga and relaxation techniques like breathing will help her get out of her own way and allow the inherent wisdom of her body to do its job. Putting herself in a safe and familiar environment, free from distractions and too many observers, will help her more easily connect to the natural process of birth.

In order to create an optimal birth experience for mother and child, it is very helpful for a woman to understand the hormonal processes of the various stages of labor, as well as during the immediate stages of bonding following birth. My dear friend, Anna Verwaal, refers to them as the perfect 'hormonal cocktail' for childbirth, breastfeeding and bonding.

These hormones are:
- Oxytocin- hormone of love
- Endorphins- hormones of pleasure and transcendence (natural opiates)
- Catecholamines- hormones of excitement (adrenaline)
- Prolactin- hormone of tender mothering and breastfeeding

When activated in their proper sequence, all of these hormones play a significant role in assisting a woman in labor and birth, keeping the parasympathetic nervous system activated during the first stages of labor and then the sympathetic nervous system for aid in pushing and delivery. When a woman's labor process is disrupted, she no longer has the full support of this natural hormonal sequence. Such disruptions may include: standard fetal monitoring, induction, administering pain relief during labor and birth, caesarean surgery, and separation of mother and baby after birth.

Oxytocin, known as the hormone of love, is released during all pleasurable activities, such as massage, hugging, sexual activity, eating, breastfeeding and bonding. During labor and birth, a woman has eight times more oxytocin receptor sites on her uterus than at any other time in her life. Oxytocin causes the rhythmic contractions of the uterus, which helps dilate the cervix, allows for the baby to be born, expels the placenta from the uterine wall, and reduces postpartum blood loss. In baby, as oxytocin levels increase and cross the placenta barrier, oxytocin enters the fetal brain to help protect the baby's brain cells when oxygen levels may lower in labor. Skin to skin and eye to eye contact immediately after birth enhances the release of oxytocin. This helps to lower stress levels and supports relaxation and bonding for both mother and child. Specifically during breastfeeding, oxytocin continues to nourish the mother and supports her to maintain a state of relaxation.

Endorphins are hormones that allow a laboring woman to enter into an altered state of consciousness, which helps her cope with the pain and intensity of labor. During labor, endorphins are released in the same gradual way they are released during any intense athletic event (for example the 'high' that comes at the end of running a marathon). The release of endorphins appropriately suppresses the mother's immune system, which otherwise could potentially treat the baby as something foreign in the body. Endorphins also facilitate the release of prolactin in the mother during labor in preparation for lactation and breastfeeding after birth. Conversely, if endorphin levels become too high in active labor they can inhibit oxytocin release, negatively impacting birth processes.

Catecholamines are the "fight or flight" hormones that all mammals produce to ensure survival. For instance, a woman who feels threatened during labor as a result of being disturbed, or who feels very fearful will release high levels of catecholamines. Particularly in the first stage of labor, this may cause labor to slow down or stop altogether, due to the diversion of blood flow to major muscle groups, resulting in less blood flow to the uterus and baby. Earlier in mammalian evolution, this disruption helped birthing mammals move to a place of greater safety before giving birth. In undisturbed labor, during the pushing stage, catecholamines release a sudden rush of energy, excitement and strong contractions that activate the fetal ejection reflex, causing the mother to want to push and the baby to be born. After birth, catecholamine levels will drop and as a result the mother may feel cold and/or shaky. A warm atmosphere, blankets, etc. are important to prevent catecholamine levels from rising again, which can inhibit oxytocin release. Since oxytocin helps with the expulsion reflex of the placenta, its decrease can increase the risk of postpartum hemorrhage. Catecholamines also surge in the baby in the late stage of labor, protecting the baby from lower oxygen levels and aiding in preparation for life outside the womb, including alertness, lung function, metabolic processes, and body temperature regulation.

Prolactin is the hormone of tender mothering. Levels of prolactin increase during pregnancy, initially decrease in labor and peak at birth. Prolactin is also the hormone of surrender, submission and breastfeeding. It helps create the bond between a mother and her baby, additionally creating a strong drive for the mother to put the needs of her baby first. Not merely a hormone of surrender and bonding, prolactin also produces 'fierce' protective behavior in lactating mammals, which explains why in nature animals are most dangerous during that time. In baby, prolactin levels are high after birth, which aids in further lung function development and body temperature regulation.

During an undisturbed labor and for an hour or so after birth, both mother and baby are suffused with this ecstatic cocktail of hormones. The release of these hormones, in their specific order and in relationship to one another, is Mother Nature's design of making childbirth as safe as possible for both mother and child. Optimizing the birth experience requires an atmosphere where a laboring woman feels safe and free to follow her own instincts and a model of care that enhances the chance of a natural birth.

THE STAGES OF LABOR

While every labor develops its own unique rhythm or pattern as waves of contractions slowly increase in frequency, the process can be distinctly divided into three stages and then recovery.

The first stage of labor can be compared to running a marathon, at times feeling like it's too much and then getting a second wind. In early labor, contractions help the cervix to thin (effacement) and gradually open (dilation) to about 4 centimeters. Many women are able to continue their usual activities during this time. In active labor, the cervix opens from 4 to 7 centimeters and contractions get substantially stronger. It is during this time that often a woman's bag of waters break, causing a gush of fluid. This will usually speed things up. The last phase is called transition, which varies from seconds to hours and is the time when the cervix opens from 7-10 centimeters and begins its 'transition' to the second stage. For most women, this is the most intense part of labor.

The second stage of labor begins when the cervix is fully dilated. As contractions continue to push the baby down the birth canal, a woman may feel intense pressure, similar to the urge to have a bowel movement, as the natural expulsive reflex causes the urge to push the baby out. The second stage ends with the birth of the baby.

The third stage of labor is the joyful union of mother holding child along with the birthing of the placenta, which could take about five to fifteen minutes after the baby arrives.

Recovery- Immediately after giving birth, a woman will still experience some aches and pains as her body begins the miraculous journey back to normal. This varies from several days to several weeks depending on whether she had a vaginal birth or a cesarean — (a surgical incision made in the abdomen and uterus to deliver the baby). She can continue to practice deep breathing through any cramps and use positive affirmations to stay relaxed and calm. Yoga postures should be avoided until she has stopped bleeding and has been given the okay from her doctor or midwife (see Once the Baby Arrives on page 84). Most babies are ready to nurse within a short period after birth. Not only does this support bonding between mother and child, but it also helps the uterus contract and decrease the amount the bleeding.

EMBRACING BIRTH OUTCOME

As much as a woman can plan for her baby's birth, there are no guarantees as to what the outcome will be. This is true whether it is a woman's first delivery or subsequent childbirth experience. The practice of yoga encourages a woman to let go of her expectations around the 'ideal' birth and learn to embrace her journey regardless of how it unfolds. For example, a woman may experience mixed emotions upon learning that she unexpectedly needs a c-section or if she had planned on giving birth naturally and instead decides she would like pain relief (such as an epidural). In whatever way her labor and birth unfold, prenatal yoga can provide valuable support.

By remaining open to the power of Shakti, she can use her breath to soften and remember that every experience is an opportunity to connect in deeper ways to herself and the greater, diverse Whole. Rather than seeing her outcome as imperfect, she may choose to celebrate her experience as 'perfect' for herself and equally Divine. Ultimately, regardless of how her baby enters the world, she can step into the threshold of motherhood with Grace.

BIRTH STORIES

Nicole Breitman/ The Birth of Reuben Aryeh Breitman

We are watching Saturday Night Live, and my water bag makes a little pop and starts leaking. Immediately I know the time I've been waiting for has come. Although it's past midnight, everyone naturally churns into action. I get up and go into the shower. Seth's sister goes downstairs, ignoring me when I say, "Oh, you don't have to fill the water pool up yet," and she gets the hose running. Within a few minutes in the shower the contractions are already very intense and I know I need to be in the pool. I go downstairs and sink into relief …ahhhh.

Judy the midwife has been called and soon she is over with her assistant Pam. My mother-in-law, sister-in-law, sister, husband and 2 kids are all in the house. Seth is in the pool with me and I ask him to push on my feet, putting pressure all down the sides, making a circuit between us. Having the pressure in my feet to focus on enables me to let go and not hold on to the pressure that is a tight ring around my belly. I use sound to open myself up, to make myself an open flowing channel for the baby to pass through. I am thinking about the baby and letting myself melt away as much as I can so that the baby can move down and out.

Finally the contractions feel different and Judy suggests it could be time to push. This whole pregnancy I read and reread birthing books, and religiously watched horrible cable TV birth shows in an effort to try to connect with the birth vibe. Since it had been 7 years since Seraphina's birth, I had tried to call upon my memories of labor in anticipation of this next birth, yet couldn't seem to find them. As soon as I start pushing, the physical memory comes right back and here I am again. I feel almost stuck; caught between two doors, in a place where I know I'm not going to be for long, but damn! Its so excruciating! The calm voice of experience that I earned from traveling through the birth dance twice before sits on my shoulder and keeps me calm and grounded with its voice of reason. "Its only a little while longer," it says. "This sucks, but it is going to be over soon and then you will have your precious baby, just let yourself go."

I am face down in the water. Although I am buoyant, I rest one hand on the bottom of the pool to support my weight. I put the fingers of my other hand up inside of me to feel the progress of the baby, and this is my asana that I stay in for a few hours. My water bag has mended itself from when it initially began leaking and it feels like a thick tough balloon. Every time I push, I feel the bag ballooning out, touching my fingers. Soon I make the decision that the feeling of pushing against this is not actually painful and actually feels good and I state this out loud, and Judy laughs and reflects back to me the lightness of my comment. Suddenly it's a party and everything is good! This goes on for a while until the balloon bursts, the baby's head moves down and I realize here we are, this is the real deal. Now it is a different sensation, now I remember Seraphina and Aiden's births and the three are one and I am endlessly in labor. The force of my muscles overtakes me and my vocal chords work in rhythm. I don't like it and just want out, but I don't dare verbalize this and lower the vibe--the voice on my shoulder calms me down and keeps me internally focused. I feel the presence of others in the room, but I stay within the circuit of Seth and I.

The power and urgency of the pushing is raw. I just want to push my baby out! Pam gives me sips of water and at some point I feel my energy lapsing and I ask for a teaspoon of honey. I hear the sounds in the room and register them, yet I don't interact unless I need to. The effort is superhuman, and with the end of each contraction I go into a deep place of reserve where I gain the strength to deal with the coming wave. I hear Judy suggest that I get into a different position, and when the next contraction is over, I just get up and move into it. There is not much conversation; a lot of unspoken work is taking place. The cd player reels on and on, making a timeless backdrop.

I push and push and push and push, and I don't feel the baby's head coming down. I start to feel a sense of desperation and think to myself, "If I was in a hospital and was offered drugs, I would definitely take them." Then, I think, "Why isn't it working? Why isn't the baby coming out?" Nobody else seems to be concerned or think there is a problem, so I don't get attached to the thought, and instead turn it into a rally cry where I psych myself up and say to myself that with this next contraction, I'm going to push the baby out. I reach down inside of myself and find all the strength in the world and push harder than ever. Over and over and over. Seth starts saying ,"Y E S, Y E S, Y E S!"

I like the encouragement and ask everyone in the room to chime in and we are all a team, everyone is cheering me and the baby on. I finally open my eyes and am pleasantly surprised to see the beautiful dawn light in the sky. My children have woken up and are beside the pool, woven into the tapestry of the birth room. Each contraction comes and goes and the baby moves down slowly, slowly. Judy helps me move into a more open position and now I am facing the ceiling, legs spread wide. The baby's head is right up against the water and my skin is thin and burning, I am pushing and the anticipation in the room is great, yet quiet and calm all at once. The baby's head is born, Judy asks me to flip over and my liquid bath helps me to gracefully spin around. I push the rest of the baby's body out and Judy in turn pushes him through my legs. I reach down and pick up my baby. He's white and vernixy and bluish and purplish and calm and peaceful. Quickly I get scared and wonder if he is okay. Again, Judy reflects a calm assurance back to me and tells me he is perfect. Seth and I hold Reuben and welcome him to the world, as our birth family holds us in timelessness until we all land.

Amanda Marra/ The Birth of Claudia Sallyann

Wednesday, July 6, I called my doctor as soon as the office opened. My contractions were nearly 2 minutes long now, but still erratically spaced. She said to go in and if I was 3-4cm, they would break my water and take it from there. I wasn't too thrilled about that, but 6 days of laboring in any capacity will bring you to the point of wanting an end in site. When I was finally brought to an exam room in the hospital, my water broke - now they couldn't send me home! This was it, it was really finally happening, I was going to have my baby! The nurses checked me and I was already 6cm. They were amazed that my body had made that progress with contractions still at times up to 12 minutes apart. This also reassured me that the work I did at home wasn't for nothing. The nurse wanted to set up my IV, and I told her no, just a hep lock. She was not thrilled with this. "Well, you know if you want an epidural, it'll take longer because they'll have to get the IV in and fluids running before they can do that," she said, with a bit of an attitude. "That's fine, I don't plan on getting an epidural, I've discussed this at length with my doctor and I've taken the hospital's required classes to use the natural birthing rooms," I replied. She sighed and set up my hep lock.

I was moved to a laboring room. The natural birthing rooms were taken, but they gave me a room with a working shower and informed my nurse of my intentions. The nurse put the monitors and blood pressure cuff on me and I told her that my doctor and I agreed on intermittent monitoring. She looked annoyed and said she would have to ask her supervisor about that. I told her that it was also talked about in the class I took at that hospital. She continued to give me a hard time about moving around saying that she couldn't get a good reading on the monitors. I told her I was fine, I knew my baby was fine; I needed to move. After talking to the OB on the floor, with whom I had thankfully met and discussed my birth, she finally agreed to let me shower, which felt wonderful.

My contractions continued to intensify. I felt like I wanted to escape my body. The labor had gone into my back and there was NO position that felt comfortable. I moved around; I moaned. It was so hot in that room - my mother and sister were fanning me while my husband massaged my back. Time simultaneously went so fast and so slow - a 2 minute contraction took an eternity to get through, but the hours of labor seemed to fly by. I asked to be checked and the OB came in - 9cm. We were almost there; I knew I was in the throws of the most difficult, but what should also be the quickest, part of my labor. It continued on with my mother, sister, and husband shifting jobs - keep me cool, keep me hydrated, keep me as comfortable as possible. A new nurse was on duty who had attended natural births, thankfully, and she was so encouraging and supportive. "You can do this, you're doing great!" It seems so simple, but hearing that when you just want to collapse holds you up. 30 minutes goes by, I still don't feel the NEED to push, but WANT to push - I want to see my baby; I want this agony to be over.

The OB checks me- 9.5. She can still feel some cervix. She explains what I already know - no pushing until 10, otherwise the cervix could inflame, making the whole process take longer. The internal battle continues. 45 minutes later, another check, still not ready. I cry. I cry a lot. I start to lose my breath, my focus; I don't know if I can do this any more. She leaves me with my family, who continue to support me, but I am scared and tired. The OB comes back in, "Amanda, I know this is not what you want to hear, and I want you to make your own decision, but you've been through a lot. I believe if you get the epidural at this point, it may allow your body to open. We'll do it light - just enough to take the edge off, and we'll turn it off as soon as you're at 10." I cave; after all, I am only human.

I get the epidural, using the support of my mother, whom they allowed to stay because she is an RN at the hospital. Getting the IV had no real affect on how long it took (even though the nurse had tried to use that as a scare tactic) because we had to wait for the anesthesiologist anyway. I lay back and feel the relief crawl into my body. Surprisingly, I don't feel good about this. "I can't believe this is how women go through labor," I tell my mother. I wanted to be an active participant - I had been, I remind myself - and will continue to be. I can still feel the contractions, but they're like a distant whisper compared to before. 40 minutes later, a final check, I'm at 10. Epi off, wait a few minutes and PUSH.

And boy did I push! I pushed on my sides, I pushed on my back, I pushed squatting using a bar, I pushed on hands and knees. My doctor and nurse were AMAZING. I pushed for nearly 2 hours and nothing. My OB stopped by the hospital to see how I was doing and told me the baby was posterior and pushing will usually turn them, but for some reason, my little girl wasn't budging. I cried again, I felt defeated again. She told me if I wanted, I could continue to push, but it could easily be a few more hours. More tears came, this is not what was supposed to happen. I had prepared, I was ready, I knew how to avoid the medical tricks and complications... and here I was, beyond exhausted. "I'm done," I told my doctor. "Amanda, I don't want you making any decisions you'll regret. You can do this if you want to." "No, Doctor, I'm done," I said through tears. The memory of this moment is the clearest of my experience. I knew I had done all I could.

Claudia Sallyann was born via emergency cesarean birth at 10:01pm on July 6, 2011. It was not how I had imagined things happening at all, but my baby was healthy and beautiful. I was told that she was malpositioned in a way that any amount of pushing I did likely would not have safely gotten her out. It took me months to come to terms with this decision, but I believe it was the right one, and I also know it was MY choice, my decision to come to - not a doctor's or spouse's, or anyone else. Claudia nursed as soon as she could and there is no weakness, or shadow of doubt of the bond I have with my daughter. I am thankful for my yoga practice and studies not only to have gotten me through my labor, but to have gotten me through my recovery. I learned how strong I was through her birth. I know that if I am blessed with a child again, I CAN do it, and I am lucky to have a doctor who has already said she would support me.

MaryJo Rosania-Harvie/ Henry's Birth Story

I prepared for labor with a series of Hypnobirth classes meant to alleviate any fears. The odd thing was, I had no fear associated with giving birth. I felt ready for it and knew exactly what to do. Because of yoga, I understood the importance of my breath and as they said in Hypnobirthing "breathing the baby down." The fears I had were related to surgery. When it came to C-section, my belief was that if I didn't let it enter my mind, it wasn't real, and it couldn't happen to me.

On my due date I went to my midwife for a stress test and, due to my gestational diabetes, a CALM score analysis. (The CALM test measures your baby's risk of shoulder dystocia in the birth process.) Two weeks prior my score was low, but now it went from low risk to moderate. Not showing any signs of labor, the midwives felt it would be at least a week until I'd deliver. If I waited the score would move to high risk. We were forced to decide right then and there to deliver via c-section, or wait. For the first 30 minutes this decision was difficult. I cried my eyes out. Then, it dawned on me. This was truly our first parenting decision. Our son was the main priority – my scar would heal, my fear of surgery paled in comparison to risking the health of our baby.

Henry would be born at 5:30 the next day. We checked in the hospital at 4:30. I held back tears as I was wheeled into the operating room, mainly due to the excitement over meeting my son! The midwife held me as the anesthesiologist administered a spinal. I used my breath to ground down on the surgical table. As I breathed, I felt a calm sensation – this was it! The OBGYN, midwife and nurses (all women!) helped me onto the table and prepped me to deliver my son. I kept focused on my breath and listened to the conversations in the room, the sound of surgical instruments unwrapped and placed on trays, monitors beeping, and the anesthesiologist's voice.

Even with the spinal, I felt the baby emerge (which did not hurt, just pressure) and felt the difference between his energy inside and outside of my body. Immediately after he was taken out I knew he was not inside anymore. I watched the doctors take him to the warmer and heard them ask my husband to "cut the cord" (which was already separate from my body – he was across the room!), then demanded they bring him to me. Someone (I can't remember who now) held my baby's face next to mine and I kissed him as many times as I could, then he left with the nurse and my husband. I get tears in my eyes when I think of that first moment when he was separate from me and not even in the same room anymore. The doctor and midwife spent the next 45 minutes putting me back together. Recovery was not easy. I couldn't hold Henry right away, but he was in the nursery bonding with his dad as he had his first bath. My husband was not sure who he should be with, Henry or I, but I assured him to stay with Henry.

Myriam Lluria Sitterson/ The Hospital First Birth

It was Friday afternoon and my house cleaner took one look at my face and said, "You're having that baby this weekend." I was very excited, and felt more than ready to give birth to my first child (didn't know the sex) by then, even though my due date was two weeks away. My former husband and I went out for Mexican food and a movie that same night. I was told the Mexican food might help move things along. In the middle of the movie I started experiencing lower back pain, which continued after I got home, about 3 hours in total. I thought for sure I was in labor, so I called the attending OB/GYN on call (there were 5 in the group) and he told me to go the hospital. As soon as I arrived they put me in a wheel chair, even though I was perfectly fine walking. I think this starts the "birth is a medical condition" mentality.

I was taken to a room, given a hospital robe and put into a bed (if you can call it that). They performed some standard procedures, stuck an IV in my arm, then checked my cervix to see how dilated I was. I was only one centimeter at that stage. I was in a lot of pain laying flat on my back, it was not at all comfortable, in fact it was agonizing! Eventually they let me get up and walk around with the IV attached, but it felt immensely better than flat on my back (a position I later learned is actually dangerous). At one point, my labor wasn't progressing to their liking, and there was an emergency C-section down the hallway. I heard a doctor yell out, "Pit her!" I was given a dose of the drug Pitocin to move the labor along. In a little bit I felt as if I were going to implode, the pain was so unbearable! They put an internal monitor on me (attached to the baby's skull) because the contractions from the Pitocin had put it into distress. Then they called in the Anesthesiologist to give me an epidural, so that I could deal with the abnormally intense contractions I was experiencing. My former husband was told to leave the room for 15 minutes, and 45 minutes later, they had not finished putting that needle into my spine! I believe it was inserted at least 5 times. When the epidural finally kicked in I could feel nothing from the waist down. I was once again flat on my back and strapped to all kinds of things. I remember being told to push and not feeling a thing. I couldn't push! So the doctor instructed me to push with all my might from wherever I was able to feel. I was then given an episiotomy, where they cut the walls of the perineum and posterior vaginal wall to make more room for the baby to come out. I don't recall exactly how long I pushed, but I thought I'd pass out from exhaustion.

When my daughter finally came out, it was 15 hours later and I was battered, bruised and in tears. I felt horrible. I told my former husband to send everyone home (family members in the waiting room), that I couldn't see anyone. My body was swollen, the blood vessels on my face had burst and there were red dots everywhere. My perineum was in agony and I could barely move. They took my baby away, gave her a pacifier and water with sugar without even asking. (I didn't have a birthing plan. I trusted my doctors 100% to take care of me and my baby.) When I tried to breastfeed, my daughter was sucking on the pacifier. My breasts became painfully engorged with breast milk. This made is almost impossible for her to latch on and excruciating for me. I had pain from head to toe and to make things worse, my former husband decided he needed to go home to get a good night's sleep, so I was left there alone. The nurses barely came in to check on me, until I was asleep, which is when they came in to check my temperature and blood pressure. I had to beg for a decongestant (I couldn't breathe through my nose) and Tylenol for the breast engorgement and throbbing pain from the episiotomy.

It was the worst experience I've ever had to date. I vowed then and there, that I would never go through that again. I also experienced severe headaches for two years after this birth. I believe this was due to the punctures in my spine from the epidural anesthesia.

Myriam Lluria Sitterson/ The Second Birth

After my first hospital birth experience, I vowed to never turn my power over to doctors, nor to trust a medical system to handle my births. I educated myself with an arsenal of birth books, my favorites by William and Martha Sears, a doctor and nurse couple who have 8 children. While I couldn't convince my former husband in favor of a home birth for the second child, we compromised and I hired a nurse midwife to handle my birth in a hospital setting, but in a birthing suite and with a birthing plan.

For starters, it was much nicer being under the care of one practitioner rather than a group of doctors, who you never really got to know and feel comfortable with. My nurse midwife was medically trained and a part of the medical system. However, the doctors created a very hostile environment for her; there were only one or two who fully supported her work.

We had asked my mother to spend the weekend at our house since we had a 22 month old and I was approaching my due date. It was a Friday night and my former husband had spent the day at a golf or fishing event (can't remember which), and he had gotten a lot of sun and was exhausted! We were laying in our bedroom and down the hall I could hear my mother singing The Twelve Days of Christmas to my daughter Carolina- it was April 25th! I went into a laughing fit and I swear that is what put me into labor. By the time I felt sure that I was having contractions, my former husband had fallen asleep saying, "Wake me up when you're really ready to go to the hospital." I was ready!! Did I mention he's my former husband? I was having a lot of lower back pain by the time we got into the car. The hospital was a 30 minute ride at most. I labored in the front seat with my feet up on the dashboard to relieve the pain. By the time we arrived at the hospital I was already four centimeters dilated! I put on my beautiful white cotton nightgown and then decided to have a shower and wash my then waist length hair. I had thought about having a water birth (had read a lot about it), but what I wanted at that moment was a hot shower. No IV, no meds and no one restricting me or telling me what to do, I entered that shower and labored under a stream of hot water, squatting when the pain became too intense for me to stand, while my former husband and the nurse midwife sat around talking and drinking coffee.

By the time I finished my shower I was 9 centimeters dilated, but that's when the pain became incredibly intense. I got dressed and my then husband began to massage my hips the way he was shown in our birthing classes. In order to check my vitals my nurse midwife put me in the birthing bed/chair. The only way I could maintain my composure was in a kneeling position and I did this for a while until she made me turn over and put my legs into stirrups (never again), which made the back pain excruciating, and then she broke my bag of water (she should not have).

My labor intensified to its peak, and I birthed my second baby, naturally!! I nursed my beautiful baby daughter while she was still attached to me via our umbilical cord. I never experienced the pain or engorging I had with my first daughter! No pacifiers, no water with sugar, no vaccines or blood tests…. that was all part of my birth plan and all went as planned, thanks to God and to my freedom to take control of the birthing process.

Myriam Sitterson/ The Third Birth - First Home Birth

After one very medically managed birth in a hospital and one birth with a nurse midwife in a hospital setting as well, I decided it was time to take things into my own hands and have a homebirth. At first, my then husband, was not keen on the idea, but knowing myself and my body as well as I do, I told him I would not put myself in the same situation I had been in with my first two births. I told him that when he gave birth he could choose where that would take place, but that I was having a homebirth the third time around. He eventually agreed to go along with my plan.

The main midwife's office was in Broward County and I went there for several prenatal appointments, and for the ones in between, I saw one of her assistants who was in Miami. I loved how relaxed and nonmedical these appointments felt. They were very professional in their approach, but also very relaxed and made me feel the same way. The assistant midwife, Nadine, was also a masseuse, and we bonded immediately. I scheduled a massage with each visit to the Miami office and very quickly decided that my main connection was with Nadine. I loved being cared for by midwives, loved how natural it felt, and how informative and gentle the appointments felt. My friends thought I was crazy to be having a home birth. My best friend said she'd pay for a stand by ambulance and I asked her to please not impose her fears on me. She had had two very unnatural and scary c-sections. She couldn't understand that I was well aware of the birthing process and wanted this birth to be as natural as possible. My second birth would have been great had the nurse midwife not insisted on laying me on my back and putting my feet in stirrups and then rupturing my bag of water. I read a lot after that birth, because everything had been going so smoothly up until the point of intervention. I wanted this third birth to be allowed to continue and evolve and happen organically.

Around 4 a.m. I started having what I recognized as contractions. I went downstairs so as not to wake my then husband, and began to prepare my daughters' lunch boxes for school. I made breakfast, all the while feeling the contractions get stronger but not unbearable. I woke the girls who were five and three at the time, got them ready for school and then woke my husband up, made him breakfast, and sent them on their way. When he returned we called the midwife and let her know I felt the birthing process had begun. Gradually and continuously the contractions became stronger and closer together. By noon I was definitely feeling some back labor. I put on some Ottmar Liebert music and started to dance in my bedroom. My midwife informed me that gyrating and moving my pelvis could help relieve some of the discomfort of the contractions. I danced and danced until I was tired of dancing, and it did in fact help. We ordered lunch from a local french bistro and my husband picked it up for all of us.

My then yoga teacher and acupuncturist, Claire Amarena, came by for a while and we lit a candle for the birth. She sat in my room and watched and encouraged me. It was a very serene setting, very natural. I wore a white nightgown and labored in my own bedroom, in the comfort of my home. In between contractions the midwives would measure my cervix. They never interrupted me, never stopped the flow of my dancing or moving around the room. It was really lovely. When the girls got out of school the babysitter brought them upstairs and together we chanted "I love you" to the new baby and "open" to my uterus. They were not alarmed at all, and were very excited to know they would soon have a new baby brother or sister. One went off to her piano class and the other to a birthday party and while they were gone, I gave birth to my third daughter. There was really no pushing, very little screaming and most importantly, no artificial intervention. Nadine, the midwife who massaged me regularly, asked if I wanted to move things along, and I did, so she applied some acupressure to my ankles to get the contractions moving along quicker. She also massaged my hips for quite a while when I was having back labor. My husband did as well. Even though it was exhausting, it was a very peaceful, beautiful and natural process. (I can almost remember it as I write this. I'm playing music that is similar to the one I played then as I write.)

At one point Nadine advised me that I was almost completely dilated and that she was going to help me by putting her hands up my birth canal, and then she did. I let out one big yell (I sounded like Barbara Streisand in one of her funny girl roles) and out came little Myriam. No tearing, no bruising! I was in an upright position when she dropped (which is how I felt comfortable in the second birth also, up until the nurse midwife intervened). No compressing on my spine, no legs in stirrups, no disharmony with my natural rhythms. It happened how I wanted it to and knew that it could. The placenta came out without a problem; Myriam latched on and nursed beautifully and

I never engorged. The midwives stayed and cleaned up the bedroom, stayed with me for several hours and left when we were comfortable and settled in with our new baby. They came back the next day and the following day. It was so different than the hospital setting. No one woke me at night to pinch and prod. No one disturbed my sleep, or took my baby away.

My pediatrician agreed to make a house call the next day, and gave little Myriam the highest apgar score. She had no jaundice. We did not vaccinate, draw blood, or do any of the things they do in a hospital. I was very content with the entire process. I felt in touch, in control and in good hands throughout the birth. I knew that if I had another baby, I would choose to homebirth again.

Tina Giazzoni-Fialko/ Rowan's Birth Story

On June 18th, my precious baby was born after quite an intense journey. My due date was June 5th. The following week of June 11th, I had an appointment with the midwife who began to talk about induction on June 19th, which would have been two weeks after my due date. My desire was to avoid Pitocin at all cost, so I began trying natural ways of moving things along. I scheduled an acupuncture appointment on Wednesday, began walking stairs, rode on bumpy roads in Chestnut Hill, ate spicy foods, walked and walked and walked, tried drumming, yoga, visualized opening and talked to my baby about coming out. I felt a little crampy on Wednesday, but the crampiness went away. I talked with the acupuncturist, who did another treatment for induction. Again I was a little crampy, here and there, but the intensity and regularity of the crampiness came and went. On Friday I had an appointment with the midwife, where they monitored the baby's heart rate and amniotic fluid to be sure that he was healthy. All was well, I was having small contractions, but they were not considered to be labor. I was one centimeter dilated, the same as I had been the previous week. The midwife asked if I would like her to separate my membranes. She did and I began to feel crampy again. I was happy. I felt things were moving along.

On Saturday morning around 3 am I awoke with definite labor pains. I called the midwife, who told me when the contractions were closer together and I was unable to talk during contractions, I should come to the hospital. Saturday was a beautiful day. My sister and husband were amazing support. We spent the day outside. I walked, did stairs, acupressure, etc, etc. My contractions became closer, then further apart, over and over throughout the day. By 11 pm, I was feeling exhausted. I was not sure if the contractions were more intense or being tired made them feel more intense. I called the midwife who told me to come to the hospital to be assessed. I was 2 cm dilated. The midwife suggested that I take Ambien, a sleep medication so that I would be able to sleep a little and have energy to push the next day. I was hesitant to this idea and asked if she could do another sweep of my membranes, hoping that might speed things up. I continued to walk the halls and stairs in the hospital, showered swaying my hips to the music, nipple stimulation, visualized opening more, certain that she would check me and I could avoid Ambien, medical interventions, etc, etc. Around 1 or 3 am, she checked me again. Nothing had changed and I decided to take the Ambien, which allowed me to sleep for a few hours.

On Sunday morning I continued with the previous evenings endeavors, confident that in time things would begin to progress. We walked outside on the beautiful grounds of the hospital where there were birds, a water fountain, native plants, an opportunity to reconnect with nature, the earth. This gave me strength to continue through the morning and early afternoon. By later in the afternoon, I was unable to keep food down. I was hopeful and relieved, thinking I was experiencing the transition. The midwife checked me and I was 2 and a half cm dilated. The only additional non-medical intervention that we all could think of was castor oil. At that point though, my body felt weak, uncomfortable and unable to handle explosive diarrhea. I took a bath in the jacuzzi tub opened myself to any possibility, medical and non-medical. My confidence that I could use only natural methods began to wain and after we talked to the midwife I decided to try Pitocin and an epidural. In retrospect, this feels sad, but I could see no other possibilities. She broke my water, began pitocin and I dilated to 6 cm. I could feel a new type of pressure and some opening in my hips. My contractions began to come closer, but after 5 units of pitocin, the baby's heart rate began to decelerate. As soon as they stopped the pitocin, his heart rate was fine, but my contractions again moved to 7 or 8 minutes apart and I didn't dilate anymore. Sometime during the evening I developed a fever, and there was meconium. They decided that a c-section was necessary.

At 8:07 Monday morning, my little love, Rowan, was born. He is amazing, healthy, adorable, and precious. My heart grows each time I hold him and each time I think of him. I'm thankful for the journey of labor that grew me in ways I don't yet comprehend. I'm thankful for the sacred experience of my entire pregnancy, the connections I developed with him along the way. I credit so much of the richness of the experience to the guidance you provided during the yoga classes. Thank you, Sue, for being a part of this journey that now continues in new directions.

Julie Pizzuti/ Roma Josephine's Birth

I began feeling surges Friday night around midnight. I felt through it for a couple of hours before telling my husband, Pat. He was so excited when I let him know our labor was beginning, his face lit up so sweetly! For over a week we'd been receiving increased pressure from our midwives to induce because our baby "was approaching 42 weeks." This was our first child, and we didn't know what to expect, but we intended on having a natural birth, with as few interventions as possible. We were seeing a group of midwives that was part of a hospital, and apparently the hospital has a policy to not let pregnancy exceed 42 weeks. I had been getting acupuncture and trying all the tricks: spicy foods, massaging acupressure points, visualizations, you name it! The surges were a welcome release of hormones to send us naturally on our way – they were relieving, exciting, and such a blessing to us! I had 1-2 surges an hour throughout the night and next day. Since labor was beginning, I was able to push off another scheduled fetal monitoring for a while, but that night they strongly urged us to come in to check the heartbeat and make sure all was well. We went to the hospital around 9pm, and were once again met with pressure to "move things along" with various induction methods. It just didn't seem right to induce when all signs pointed to a healthy baby – still lots of amniotic fluid, no signs of fetal distress, perfect heart rate, etc. The only reason given for induction was that I was believed to be approaching 42 weeks based on an estimated due date (and I think the fact that it was a holiday weekend had something to do with it as well – the staff was anxious to get things wrapped up). This time, because we refused induction, we had to sign several legal statements indicating that we were made aware of the potential risks involved with refusing induction. The midwife apologized, and said it was a policy to protect the doctors from potential litigation. I asked, had we chosen to induce, would we have had to sign similar documents indicating our understanding of the risks involved with induction. The answer was no.

We went home around 10:30pm, and at midnight I began feeling strong surges, 5 minutes apart, lasing about 60 seconds each. My water broke around 1:00 am, and soon my surges were 3 minutes apart. Pat was getting nervous and trying to coax me into the car to go to the hospital. We had been employing the Hypnobirthing techniques we'd been practicing, and I was doing well finding comforting breaths during surges, then relaxing in between. I was reluctant to disturb my state of mind by getting in the car. I also kept thinking that we had so much time before the birth, and was mentally preparing myself by repeating "this is a marathon, not a sprint!" When we arrived at the hospital at 4am I was 8cm dilated. I was surprisingly calm though my surges were strong now and 2 minutes apart. I was wheeled into our birthing room and Pat began setting up all the flameless candles we brought. I had envisioned a dimly lit roomful of candles to greet our new baby. I had decided early on to be excited, not afraid, about the birth, and thought about our hospital stay as if we were going to a bed and breakfast — after all, we were the customers, so we should have things the way we wanted them, right? I wore my own comfortable night gown during my labor and birth. I had made a delicious vegetable broth and brought snacks in case I needed them (though I had to say they were for my husband because I was only allowed clear liquids once admitted). I had beautiful music, my favorite essential oils for aromatherapy, a bathing suit for the tub, my favorite tea, my yoga mat, tennis balls for Pat to massage my back, a knotted scarf to hang from if I felt the urge — we even brought a bottle of my favorite wine! Two hours after we arrived at the hospital our beautiful 7lb 13 oz daughter, Roma Josephine, was born into a roomful of soft white candlelight — I didn't even have time to use any of the goodies we brought! I was so into my breath and surrendering my mind to the innate intelligence of my body that the thought of pain medication never occurred to me. Feeling the surges and breathing down my baby was the wildest, most primal experience I've ever had. Something sacred took over to guide this process, and I felt like an observer watching my body do exactly as it needed to do. I will never forget how amazing and powerful I felt as her head emerged, and how clearly I could feel her body moving through mine — an experience I could not have had being numbed with medication. She was so bright and alert. She was immediately placed on my chest upon entering the world, and sniffed her way to my left breast to nurse. Having a generally low tolerance for pain, I was shocked that I didn't need so much as a Motrin, even in the weeks following her birth.

As it turned out, after some initial standard measurements were taken, our midwife said Roma was probably less than 41 weeks — not over 42 as was conveyed to us earlier. It goes without saying that we are so glad we waited for our daughter to come to us on her own, and proud of ourselves for resisting the pressure to induce. We had a simple birth plan that we communicated to the midwives and labor nurses ahead of time and they respected our requests, such as not using erythromycin on her eyes, letting the cord stop pulsing before cutting it, and letting Pat announce the sex of the baby to me. We had a truly divine and beautiful experience overall, proving that it is possible to have a comfortable, natural hospital birth (even in a hospital with very high epidural and c-section rates) — if you know how to ask for it.

Jennifer Skelton/ Dylan's Birth Story

With my first son Jordi I had tried for a completely natural childbirth. As a yoga teacher with prenatal training and a keen interest in childbirth, I had read lots of books and had a good understanding of the process of labour and childbirth.

Since I live in a remote part of Canada — the city of Yellowknife in the Northwest Territories — I do not have access to home birthing midwifery services. The hospital has a team of 10 or so family doctors that attend births and take turns being on call. Unfortunately there is no way to choose the doctor that will be present at the birth. For this reason, my partner Marc and I prepared a birth plan to let hospital staff know our desire for a natural birth and our specific preferences.

Labour began with strong back pain associated with contractions and no ability to rest. We laboured at home for 16 hours or so and used relaxing breath work to keep my throat relaxed while Marc helped me cope with the back labour using a rocking chair. I was 4 cm dilated when we got to the hospital and they gave us the privacy we requested while I dilated the rest of the way. Then my contractions stopped. I was exhausted and wanted to rest.

After a short rest the doctor suggested breaking my water to get labour started again. This failed to work and I was told that the longer I went without contractions the less likely they would come back on their own. I ended up being augmented with oxytocin and although I never felt an "urge to push" I was directed to forcefully push while holding my breath.

I tried various squatting and other natural positions but I was so exhausted that my arms and legs trembled and I was unable to hold them. In the end I was on my back with my knees bent into my chest and my feet pushing on a squatting bar above the bed. The forceful pushing felt awful and totally unnatural. I tore my pelvic floor badly and was uncomfortable walking or sitting for a long time after the birth. A year later I developed a stage 1 cystocele (bladder prolapse) after taking up running without fully regaining strength in my pelvic floor.

The doctors said I would need surgery to repair the cystocele once I was finished having children. I immediately began to seek out alternative sources of information. I was angry, as I knew that childbirth was a natural process and my injuries could have been prevented. I questioned the recommendations I had been given in the hospital and I researched alternatives. I was determined to learn from the experience, regain strength in my pelvic floor, and not let any future childbirth follow the same course.

I spoke with midwives across the continent and learned that there were other opinions on what to recommend when a woman's contractions stop during labour. I visited specialized postpartum physiotherapists and learned how to regain strength in my pelvic floor, minimize the symptoms of the prolapse and avoid surgery. I took additional prenatal yoga training with Sue Elkind and Anna Verwaal (a very experienced and inspiring doula). I read books and learned more about natural childbirth and methods of breathing the baby out. I was determined to understand the connections between the breath, intra-abdominal pressure, the muscles of the pelvic floor and the abdominals. I wanted to understand how it was possible to breathe the baby out with only the natural expulsion reflex of the uterus.

When I became pregnant again we hired a fabulous doula and were excited to have additional support for our next labour. My biggest fear had to do with not knowing which doctor would attend my birth and how it could affect my labour if it were someone resistant to our birth plan requests. I began to secretly visualize the baby coming so fast that we couldn't make it to the hospital!

My labour again began with strong back labour. Our doula was out of town due to a family emergency so we were once again without support. She had shown Marc how to give me a double hip squeeze with me on all fours to help alleviate the back pain while opening the pelvis and helping the baby into a more optimal position. After a few trial and error attempts we got into a groove with Marc giving me the hip squeeze for each contraction. I stayed on all fours between contractions determined that this time we would turn the baby into a more comfortable position and then REST during early labour to prepare for what lay ahead.

Without the doula, Marc found himself needing 10 hands. He was running around cooking dinner for Jordi, phoning friends that were on call for Jordi, setting up a playpen in another room (Jordi still slept in a crib in our bedroom where I was labouring), and checking on me every so often to give me a double hip squeeze.

Jordi, our two-and-a-half-year-old son, was an absolute sweetheart! He climbed up on our bed where I was on all fours and helped rub my back in between contractions while Marc was running around doing everything else. He even tried to give me a double hip squeeze after watching Marc do it! Then he agreed to go to bed about an hour and a half before his usual time with no fuss so that daddy could help mommy with the new baby.

With Jordi in bed, Marc continued giving me the double hip squeeze for each contraction. We were both hoping it might help me out of back labour at some point so we could rest but we were also preparing mentally for the possibility that this early labour would go on for as long as last time.

What we didn't realize was that this was not early labour! I was in active labour the whole time and my cervix must have dilated earlier in the day without me realizing it! So instead of realigning the baby position to help me get out of back labour, relax, and dilate better (I could feel the baby moving when he did the hip squeeze), we must have been opening the birth canal and moving the baby into it!

I got into the tub at one point to relax on my side and then started feeling a whole lot of pressure in my pelvis (like the next uterine surge would be difficult to hold off "pushing"). This was my first realization that it might not be early labour. I asked Marc to check me, as I didn't feel I could get in the car to go to the hospital. I felt I needed to pee yet couldn't pee and the pressure was intense. Marc saw no sign of the baby but reported that I was very open.

Shortly after that my water broke and it relieved the pressure somewhat but the contractions started coming quickly. Marc was still giving me pressure on my raised hip during the contractions but I asked him not to touch me no matter what. My pelvis took on a life of its own and moved wildly back and forth in the tub during the next couple of contractions. I focused on keeping my throat relaxed with the breath so that my pelvic floor would stay relaxed.

There was a short period of relief and I got on all fours again and asked Marc for another double hip squeeze. "I see the head," he said. My emotion upon hearing those words was a mixture of elation at the realization that my wish had come true and we were about to have a home birth, excitement that labour was not going to last for 30 hours again, and shock that I had not been consciously aware of what stage of labour I was in.

"Well I guess we're not going to the hospital," I said. "Get ready to catch the baby!" Marc got ready. He gave me another double hip squeeze with the next contraction while I focused on staying relaxed and calm. I took a deep breath and allowed my uterus to do its job. I felt the urge to take one hand to my belly and push it up and as soon as I did this Marc reported that the head was out. The contraction ended and Marc was looking down at a little blue head facing him with eyes closed and no movement. It must have been a little disconcerting for someone that hadn't seen that before. He was trying to stay calm, as he knew if he expressed fear it could affect me in the labour. "So, right now there is just a head," he calmly stated, "I think we need to get the body out so the baby is not being cut off at the neck." I knew it was normal for the body to come out on a subsequent contraction. I told Marc I needed to wait for another contraction, as I wasn't going to force the baby out. "Maybe if we could get you into a squatting position it would help," he said. I said I could do that so I stood up in the tub and bent my knees a little. I think I pulled my belly in slightly with the next contraction and then I heard Marc say "That's it. The baby is out and it's a boy!"

I turned around and Marc handed me the baby. He was blue and didn't make any movement or sound. After a moment he let out a little wheezing cough and then went back to being limp in my arms. I knew he was still getting oxygen through the umbilical cord but that the fluid in him also needed to come out. As he was born only about ten minutes following our realization that we were not in early labour, we were still in a bit of shock and not thinking clearly. One of us could have used our mouth to suck out the fluid from his nose and mouth but it didn't occur to us at the time. I was also standing there with the placenta not yet out and blood running down my legs (there had been no bleeding at all until after the birth). I didn't know how I would get into the car in that state to go to the hospital. We decided to call the ambulance.

The paramedics showed up just as I was getting ready to lie down to birth the placenta. It was an interesting scene with four paramedics all in full winter gear and boots walking into my bathroom where I was holding my baby while standing in a bath full of bloody water. I didn't care since I had already had my natural home birth. The only thing was that it stalled the placenta birth and I had to get oxytocin by IV when I got to the hospital in order to help my uterus expel the placenta and avoid a possible postpartum hemorrhage. It may have been unnecessary as the placenta came out soon anyway but it wasn't a big deal. I felt great and had no pain and went home the next day.

Marc and I were thrilled that we had the opportunity to experience a wonderful, natural home birth. Baby Dylan was born at about 9:25pm into his daddy's arms on October 30th, 2012, a day after the full moon. From the time we realized I was in labour it was less than three and a half hours to the birth. We worked together to help me stay relaxed and calm so that the natural expulsion reflex of my uterus could birth our baby. I never pushed and never bore down. There was no tearing. Our family bonded over the experience and Jordi absolutely loves being a big brother to beautiful little Dylan.

Stefanie Zimmermann/ Noah Narayan

Reflecting back on my boy's arrival, I can truly say it was one of the most profound, spiritual and shifting moments I have ever experienced.

My understanding of life has kept me coming back to Source, back to nature and it's most profound energies. I witnessed my pregnancy from this perspective and it literally showed me the way. Initially though, after not slowing down as my body indicated me to do and pushing too hard physically, I experienced bleeding in my first trimester. From this experience I learned to pay attention to my body more closely and to foster what was most optimal for the baby. I promised to let my inner source be my guide.

I was feeling great in my 2nd trimester and had tons of energy to 'get it all done.' Then I discovered my cervix length was below average. Rest and engaging the pelvic floor did not change this fact about my cervix, so with the risk of a premature arrival, I was placed on bed rest and received a cervix support ring. Being a physical person and identifying with that all of my life, it forced me to dig deeper. It was not only a phase of letting go of parts of my old life, but also a phase of making the soil ready for new beginnings. Luckily, it was also the start of a regular meditation practice. My meditation practice began with strong resistance, but continued into deeper peace and allowed me to cultivate new priorities. I reflected on the name Noah, which means "the peaceful one." Since the first date between my spouse Elijah, his father, and I, his name had been discussed and out there, waiting for our baby.

Patience is not exactly my strength and the two weeks Noah went past his due date felt like torture. But deep inside I knew he was fine and told myself he was just getting ready. I did my best to keep it together in the midst of many "false" labor alarms. Going in for the fifth check after my due date, I started to get upset and desperate- it was time for him to come out! I could not do this any longer. Fortunately, the midwife at the clinic who checked me took my concerns seriously and mentioned that when she was working in Africa, babies died from being in the womb too long. The placenta has a certain life span and after that span, the cells start to die. It was the story I needed to hear to feel empowered in my state. She checked me and I was 2 cm dilated; if labor was not going to get started within the following 12 hours we agreed to induce labor. Feeling carried and supported with her warm and positive words and a homeopathic "labor kickoff cocktail," I left to go home.

Elijah, who is usually the grounding force in our relationship, was restless like a cat in a cage. I escaped into the always soothing shower- my place of comfort during these last 9 1/2 months. One minute later the first contractions kicked in. Having just long enough of a break to tell him, "We need to leave for the clinic now," the contractions and muscle shaking came on like an explosion. Somehow, with his help I made it out of the shower, into the car and 15 minutes later (the ride usually takes 40 minutes), into the warm and home-like birthing room at the Paracelsus Clinic. It was 8:30 PM. The midwife on shift led me through breaks in between contractions and about 40 minutes later, while I was in the water of the tub, longer breaks between contractions set in. Fully in the zone, focusing on breath, surrender and releasing sounds, I was fully dilated by around 11:30 PM. Sometime before that my water did break. With the urge to push, still in the water and positioned on my knees, things started to slow down. As my intuitive strength started to wane, the suggestions of Elijah and the Midwife helped to move things forward. I found myself on my knees on the floor, but this didn't work. Somehow I was carried onto the bed and made my way into a squat, pushing with all my strength while holding onto the wonderful people supporting me. The releasing sounds did not work anymore to move me forward, and I was advised to push while keeping the sound in - that is when things started to move again. By 1 AM, Noah's eyes and nose peaked outside. Elijah told me later that in that moment Noah was fully present - his eyes opened, his nostrils fully expanded and as he took a deep breath and with a last push, he was fully presented. Right away he got to rest covered in warm blankets on my tummy. Time stood still. No one spoke. It was everything.

While Noah was on my tummy the doctor and the midwife took care, waited for the placenta to follow and stitched me up where I was injured. At one point the midwife intuitively pushed on my tummy and a rush of extra blood came out. Although it was very uncomfortable, what came out prevented me from potential afterbirth complications later. Waking up the next morning, looking right into the face of this perfect being, feeling each other's warm breath, I could not have wished -ever- for anything else.

ONCE THE BABY ARRIVES

Just when a woman thought the marathon was over, welcome to the 4th trimester! Life with baby in arms is certainly more joyous than labor and delivery, but that doesn't mean the first few months postpartum is not seriously challenging as well. Hormonal shifts, which happen immediately and continue the first couple of weeks, can create emotional swings and physical discomfort. Some common things a woman might experience postpartum are:

- Night sweats — as excess water is released from the body.
- Sore breasts — as milk production increases.
- Leaky breasts — if a woman chooses to nurse.
- Hair loss — which usually subsides after 6 months.
- Vaginal soreness — try soaking in sitz baths (a plastic bowl that fits over the toilet seat) and applying frozen pads soaked in healing herbs (only for vaginal births, not c-section).
- Vaginal discharge — blood flow like menstruation (lochia), which should decrease each day.
- Contractions — first few days after birth, similar to menstrual cramps, may increase during nursing.
- Skin changes — blood vessels in face may have increased during the pushing phase (these should gradually fade).
- Hemorrhoids — try soaking in sitz baths (see above) and applying cool compresses.
- Lack of sleep — due to baby's feeding schedule. Sleep when the baby sleeps.
- Leaky bladder — when sneezing or laughing. Do kegels (see page 29).
- 'Baby blues' — onset may occur during the first couple of weeks.
  Note: Some new mothers still experiencing the 'blues' beyond the second week may be one of the 10-20% of women who develop postpartum depression, a serious condition which may require medical attention.

I advise new mothers to do their best to stay home the first six weeks after delivery (offered to me by Gurmukh Khalsa and the Sikh community), which helps the body recover strength and avoid relapsing later in the year. It also allows for essential bonding time between mother and baby as they establish their new rhythm together (which is generally feeding, sleeping, and pooping!). While not all women have the luxury to spend six weeks nesting (especially if it's not their first baby), it is important for new moms to remember to take extra care and not try to be 'super mom.' If a woman doesn't have sufficient help from family members, there are postpartum doulas available to help prepare nourishing meals, clean, tend to the baby while mommy sleeps, and do laundry. New mothers having problems or new to nursing can contact La Leche League (llli.org), which offers incredible support and encouragement.

If a woman was able to stay in good shape during her pregnancy and had a healthy vaginal delivery, she can begin light exercise (walking, gentle yoga) within a couple weeks of her delivery. For a c-section, she should wait six to eight weeks to exercise, except light walking which is actually beneficial after a couple of weeks. Most doctors advise waiting until after the six week check-up before resuming a normal exercise routine. Regardless of when a woman decides to start, she needs to remember to go slowly. Her joints and ligaments will still be loose for about three to five months, so she should keep any exercise low-impact and focus on toning and lightly stretching.

Also, it is very common for a woman's abdominal muscles to separate (diastasis recti) during pregnancy or birth. It can take months for the gap to close depending on a woman's genetic history and physical condition. If she begins rectus abdominis 'crunches' before the gap is three finger widths or less, she may risk injury. (A way to check the abdominals is to lie flat on the back with the knees bent. On an exhale, lift the head and shoulders, reaching one arm towards the knees to tighten the muscles. Place fingers right above the belly button and see how wide the space is from the center out.)

POSTNATAL YOGA

A woman can immediately begin strengthening her pelvic floor muscles after birth by regularly practicing kegels. This will bring more blood flow to the pelvic region and potentially heal tears, or an episiotomy faster. Even if she has had a cesarean birth, her pelvic floor muscles have been stretched from the weight of her baby and uterus. Kegels can help!

She can also connect to her transverse abdominals right away through belly breathing, focusing on drawing her belly backwards towards her spine on her exhalations. At first this will feel very difficult and she may want to 'splint' her abdominals to help. (For instance, she can wrap a scarf around her mid-back and then pull it in front, with her right hand holding the left side of the scarf and left hand the right side of the scarf. Crossing the scarf in front of her body, she can firmly pull the scarf in opposite directions, tightening it around her abdominals for support.) Even post c-section, a woman should begin gentle belly breathing as soon as possible. This will help increase circulation around the wound which promotes healing. Activation of the abdominal muscles will also help the scar heal with increased mobility.

A woman should wait at least six weeks to start a postnatal yoga practice, if she had a vaginal birth, and eight to twelve weeks if she had a cesarean (to let the incision heal). In addition to focusing on practicing kegels and strengthening the transverse abdominals, after birth a woman should also focus on restoring her body. She can enjoy a supported savasana (placing a rolled blanket underneath her scapulas) while her baby sleeps, visualizing every cell in her body being recharged.

Once she is ready to practice, it is nice to begin at home, trying a few familiar poses that she was doing while she was pregnant. The most important thing for her to remember is to keep her transverse abdominals engaged, particularly during transitions! Starting with simple ujjayi breathing and warm-up poses, such as a tadasana and uttanasana, she can ease her way into a few different categories of poses. This will give her an awareness of where her body is in terms of strength and to what extent she is able to move and support herself with good alignment. Then she can begin to add poses that specifically build strength, like wall squats. With strong attention on integrated action in poses like down dog, plank and chaturanga, she can begin to build strength in the arms, legs, back, and abdominals. When she is ready to venture to class, postnatal or mommy and me classes are great first options and can be reassuring. Bringing baby to class is a wonderful solution to being able to practice and stay together. New mothers can also connect with each other and share similar problems and experiences. If there are no specialty classes available, she should try a beginner yoga class first and let the instructor know she is a new mom.

Benefits of practicing postnatal yoga:
- Regain physical strength
- Support overall health and well being
- Release tension in neck and shoulders
- Alleviate physical discomforts
- Replenish energy levels
- Decrease emotional rollercoaster
- Balance stress of being a new mom
- Reconnect to self
- Optimize posture
- Promote relaxation
- Rejuvenate the mind

Common postnatal issues that yoga can help alleviate:
- Weakened pelvic floor (kegels)
- Weakened abdominals (transverse abdominal work)
- Aching neck and shoulders (upper back openers and strengtheners)
- Sacroiliac pain (supta padangusthasana)
- Lower back pain (tadasana with block)
- Loss of endurance (warrior poses)
- Fatigue (legs up the wall)
- Weak gluteus (squats)
- Postpartum 'blues' (breathwork)

Most importantly, a woman should be kind to herself regardless of how much or how little she is able to do. With all of the enormous changes taking place during her '4th trimester,' including lack of sleep and a brand new life with her little one, there is everything to be proud of and celebrate. Soon enough things fall into place and new routines allow for more personal time. The sweet connections made in the quiet hours when a mother and her baby are communing with the moon are some of the most powerful moments of a woman's life.

YOGA SEQUENCES

The following yoga sequences are meant to support the different levels of prenatal yoga practitioners, ranging from beginner to intermediate. They are designed as a template and can be modified according to a woman's needs and abilities. Specific sequences for nausea, restoratives, and infertility are included. In order to avoid strain or possible injury to herself and her growing baby, it is important for a woman to take extra care not to push herself beyond her current level of yoga experience while she is pregnant. For all women, I recommend focusing on the breath and proper alignment, gently opening the body and maintaining strength (see Essentials for a Healthy Prenatal Yoga Practice, page 22). Working with an experienced yoga teacher is always advised, especially for beginners.

Warm Up/Sun Salutations

This routine can be done as a warm-up for a longer practice or simply as a sweet way to 'salute the sun' each new day.

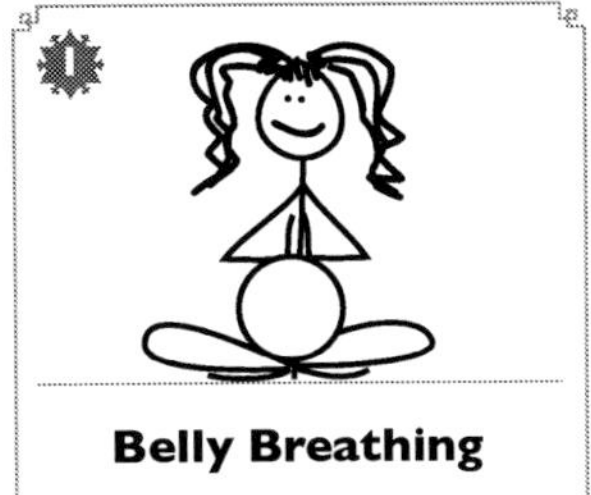

Belly Breathing

Engage the belly backwards toward the spine on exhalation. 10 deep breaths.

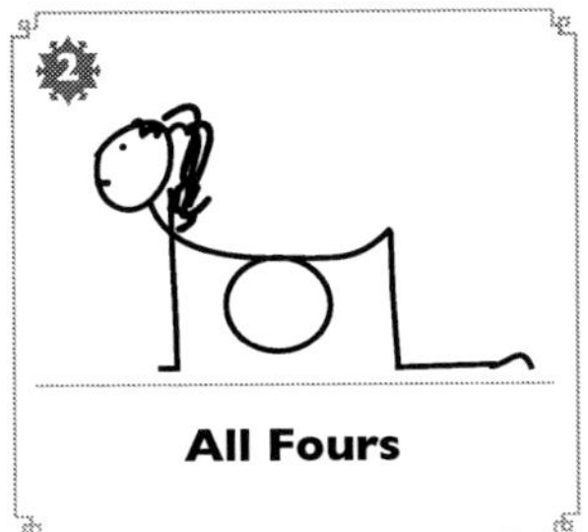

All Fours

Root hands, strengthen arms, soften heart.

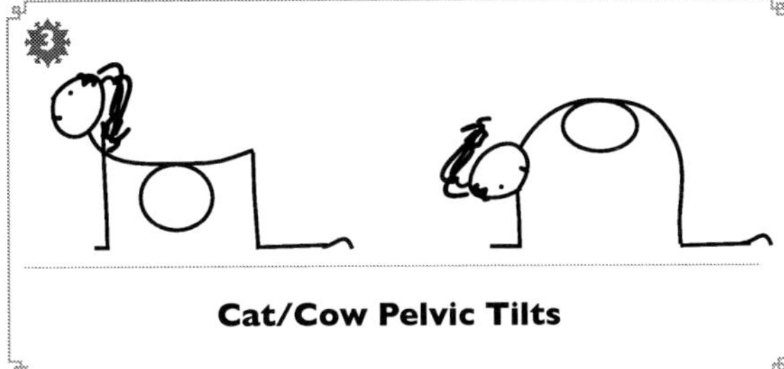

Cat/Cow Pelvic Tilts

5x. Link breath with movement; don't over arch lower back.

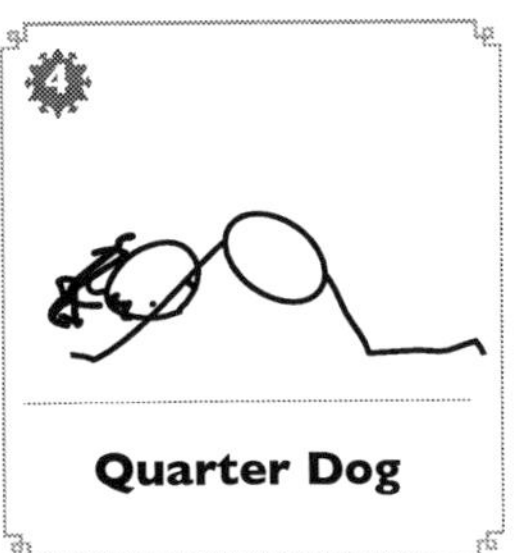

Quarter Dog

Knees on floor, arms angled back, arm bones lift.

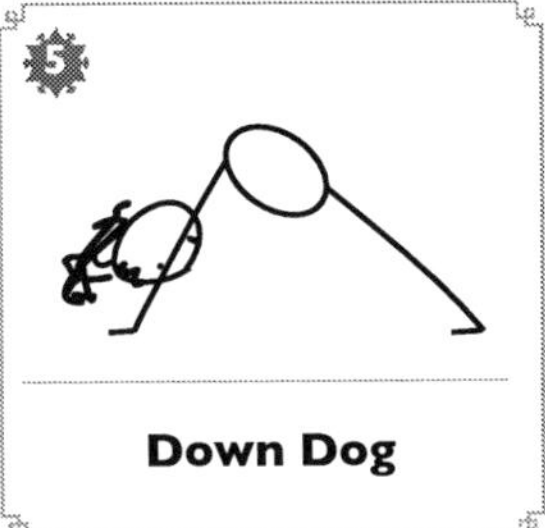

Down Dog

Wide legs, walk feet out.

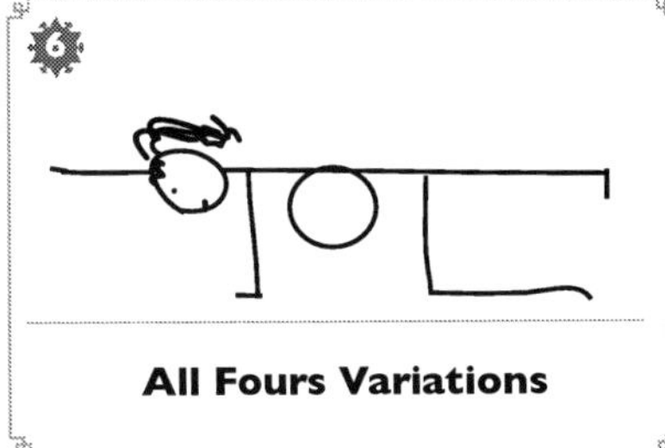

All Fours Variations

Balancing opposite arm/leg.

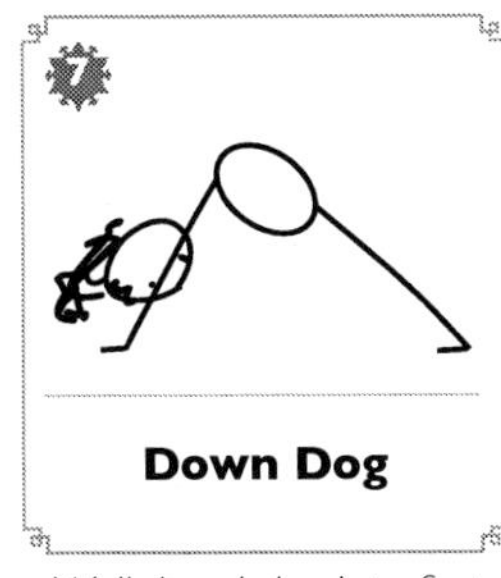

Down Dog

Walk hands back to feet for Uttanasana (standing forward fold).

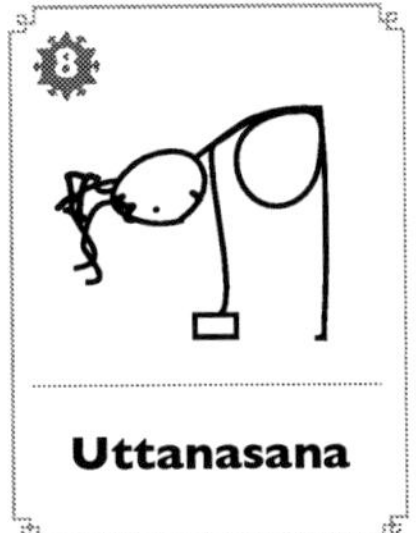

Uttanasana

With hands elevated on blocks if needed, feet wide.

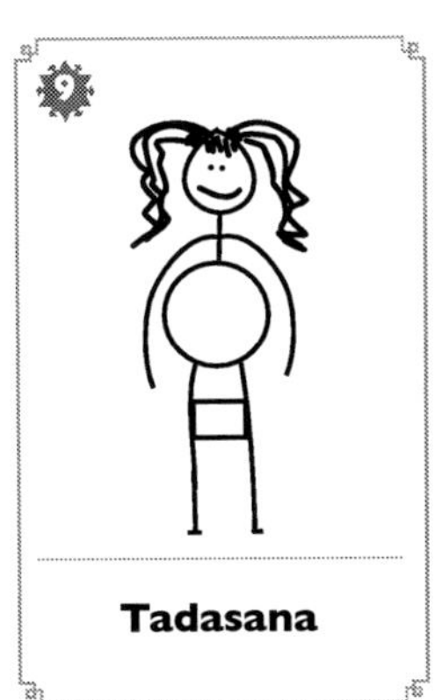

Tadasana

With block between inner thighs.

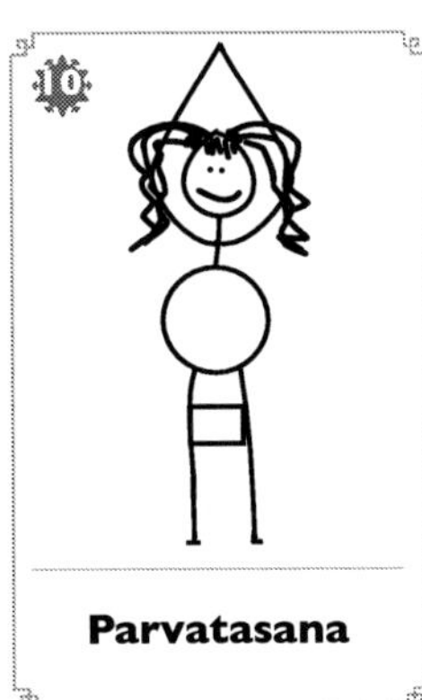

Parvatasana

Arms overhead.

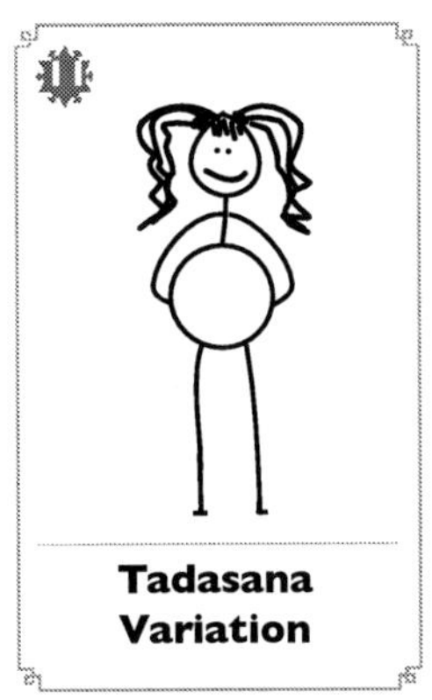

Tadasana Variation

Bound hands/shoulder stretch.

...continued on next page

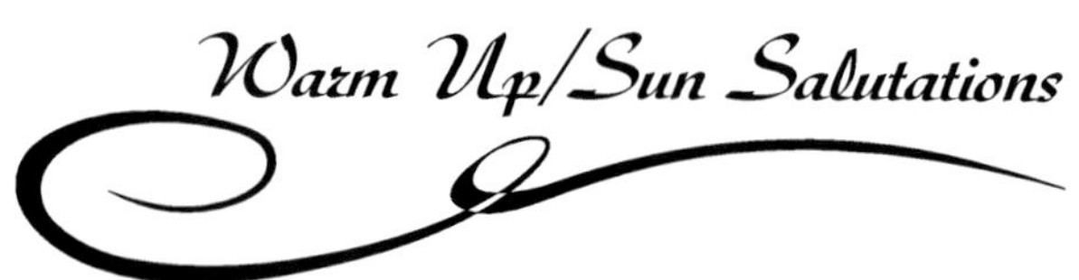

Warm Up/Sun Salutations

...continued from page 89

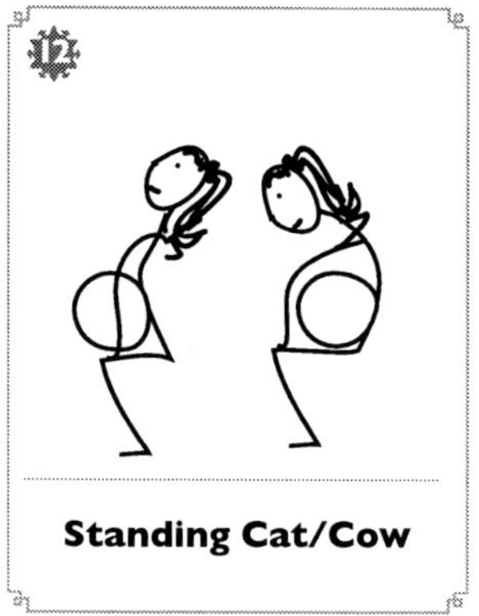

Standing Cat/Cow

Pelvic tilts.

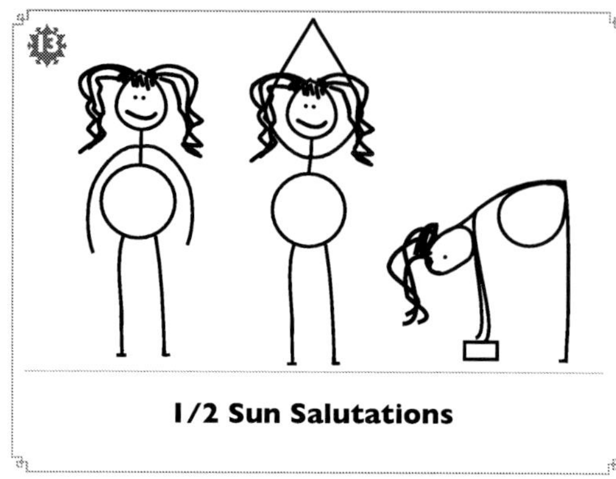

1/2 Sun Salutations

3x. Hands on blocks if needed.

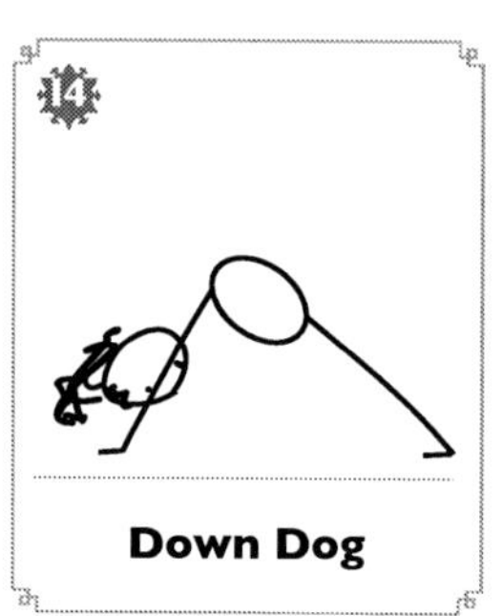

Down Dog

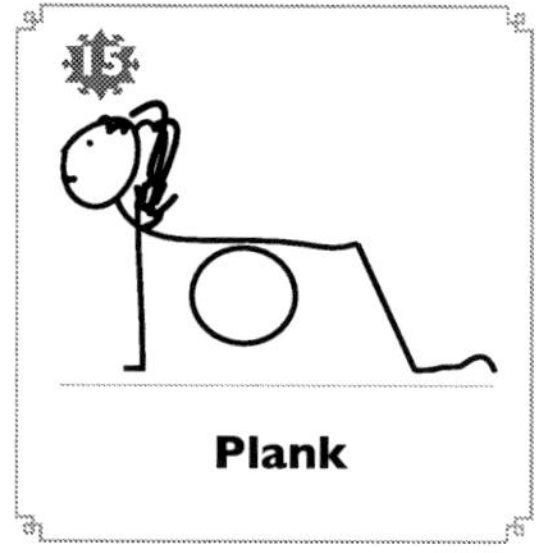

Plank

With knees on floor behind hips.

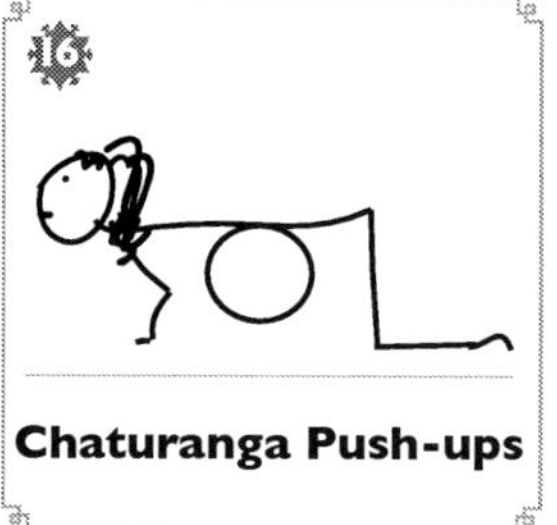

Chaturanga Push-ups

3x. Knees on floor.

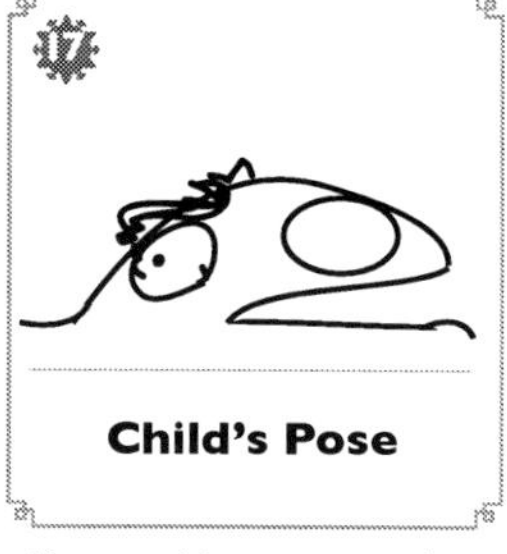

Child's Pose

Knees wide, toes together, arms forward.

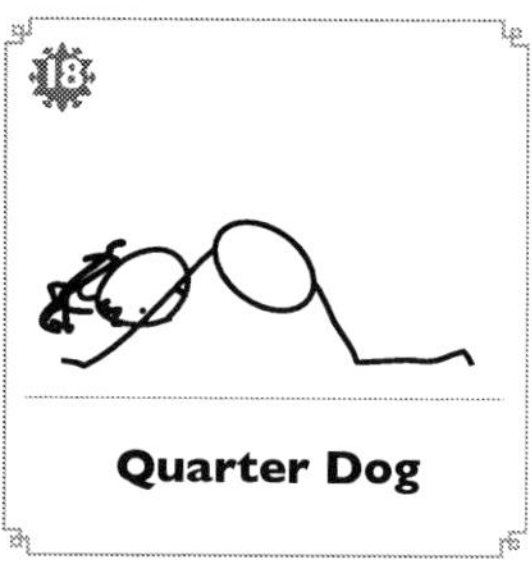

Quarter Dog

Knees on floor.

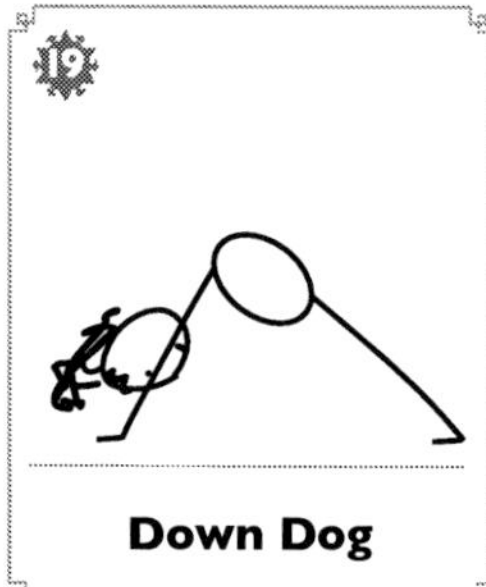

Down Dog

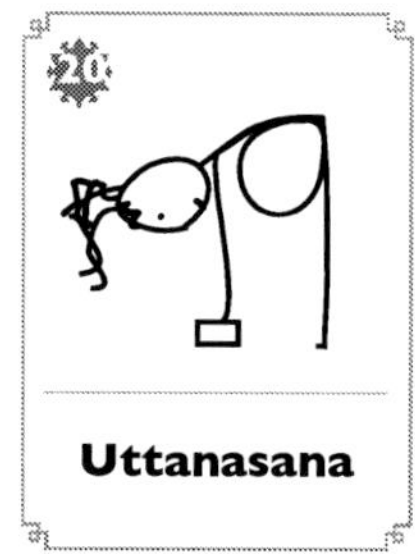

Uttanasana

With hands elevated on blocks if needed, feet wide.

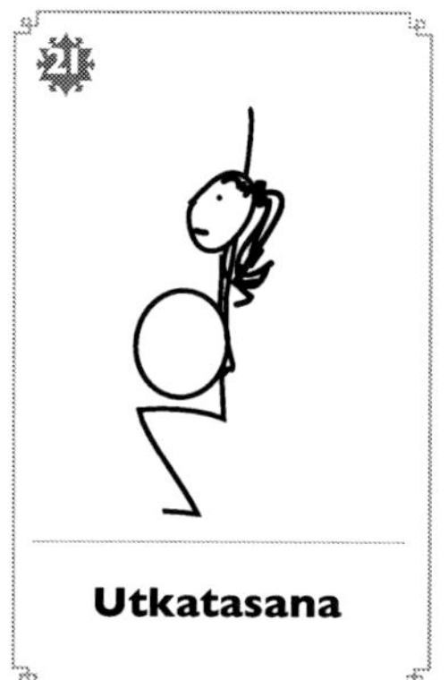

Utkatasana

To modify: either forearms to thighs, arms straight forward, final stage arms up.

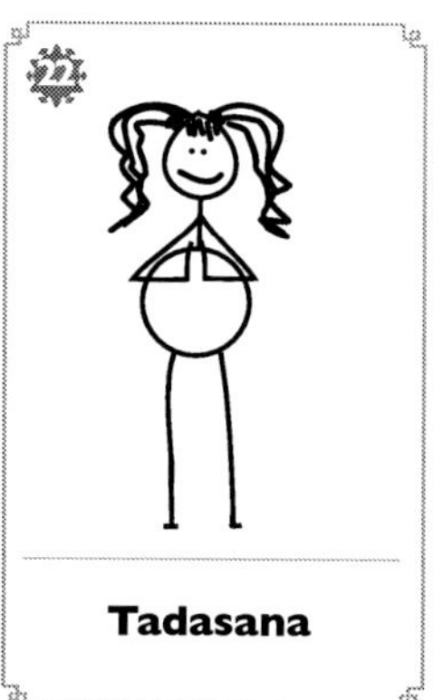

Tadasana

End with 5 deep breaths.

Beginner Sequence

This beginner sequence is safe to do regularly — supporting strength, flexibility, and balance. Note: new students should still seek a teacher to ensure proper alignment.

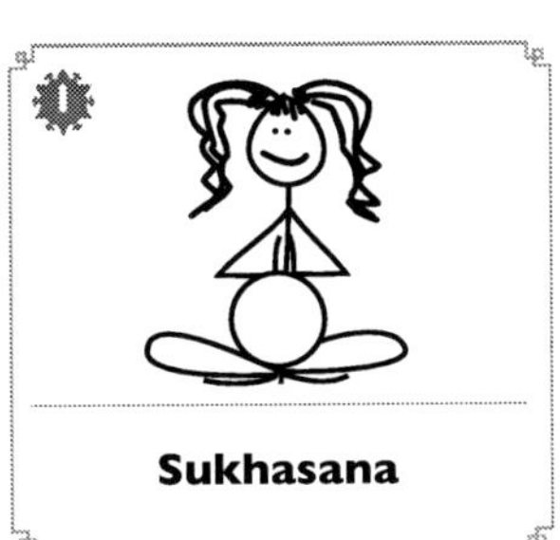

Sukhasana

On blanket for opening meditation.

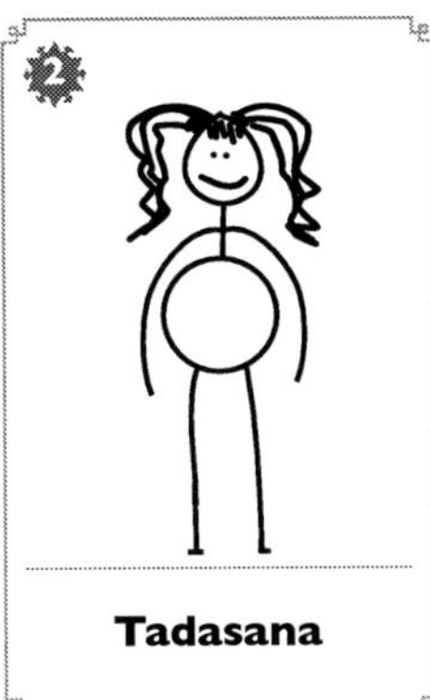

Tadasana

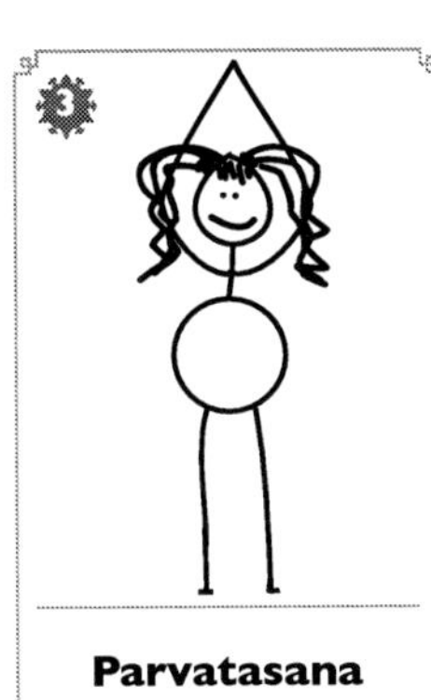

Parvatasana

Arms overhead.

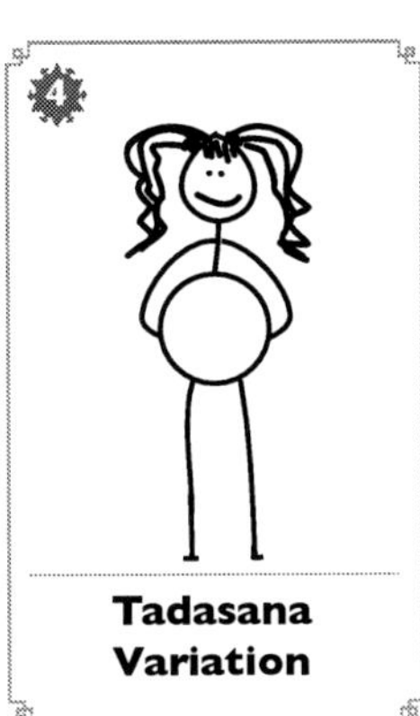

Tadasana Variation

Bound hands/shoulder stretch.

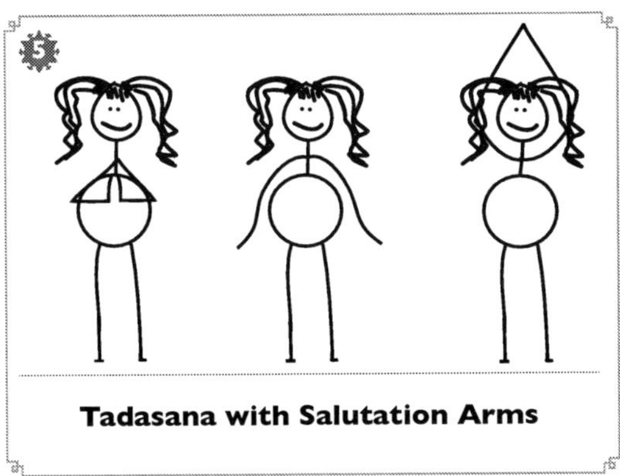

Tadasana with Salutation Arms

5x. Move arms up and down with breath.

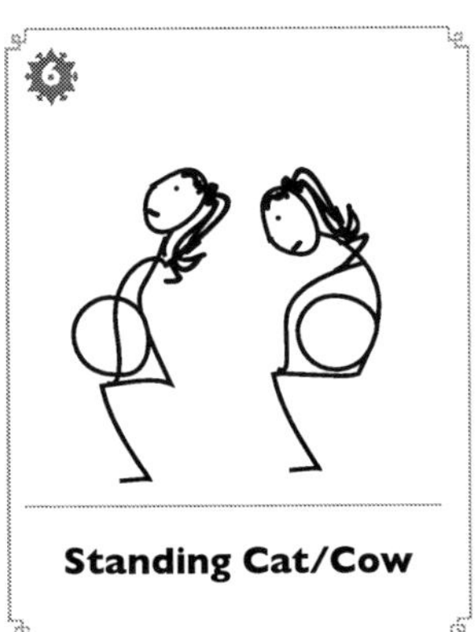

Standing Cat/Cow

Pelvic tilts.

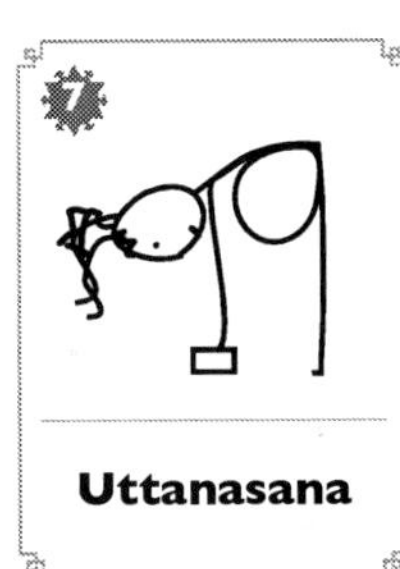

Uttanasana

With hands elevated on blocks if needed, feet wide.

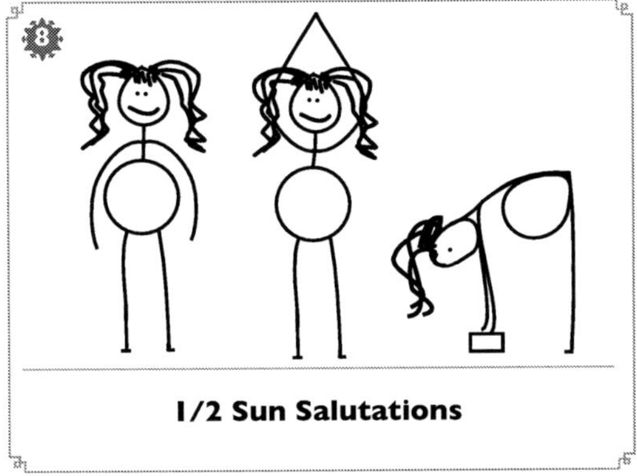

1/2 Sun Salutations

3x. Walk arms forward to all fours.

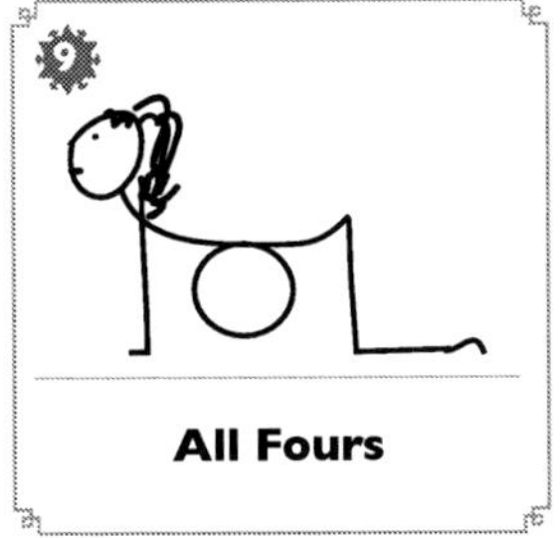

All Fours

Root hands, strengthen arms, soften heart.

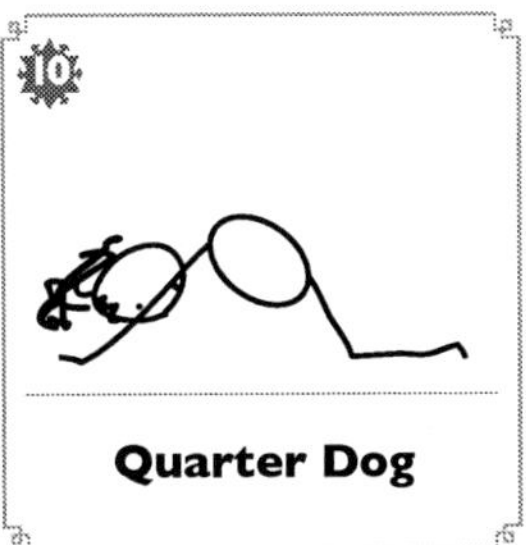

Quarter Dog

Knees on floor, arms angled back, arm bones lift.

...continued on next page

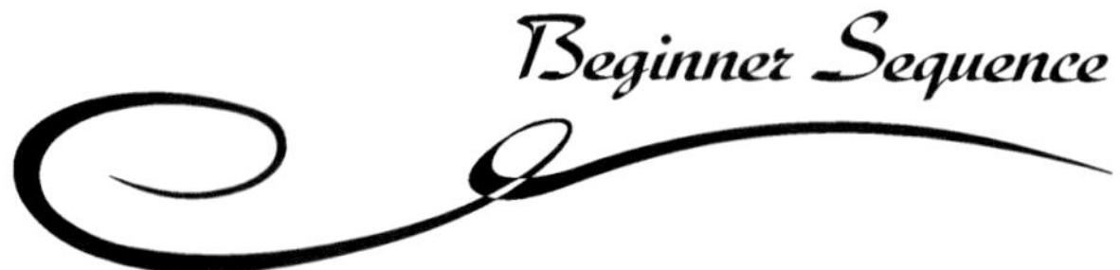

...continued from page 91

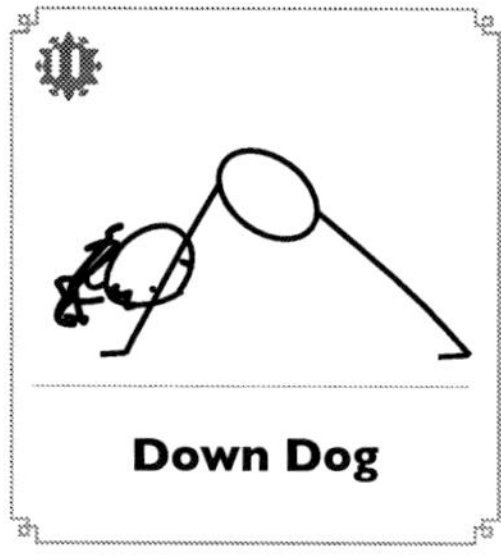

Down Dog

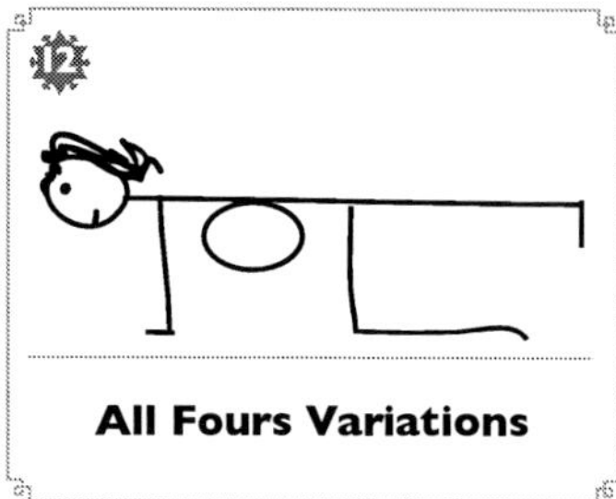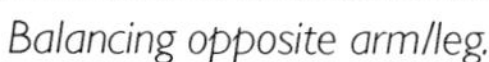

All Fours Variations

Balancing opposite arm/leg.

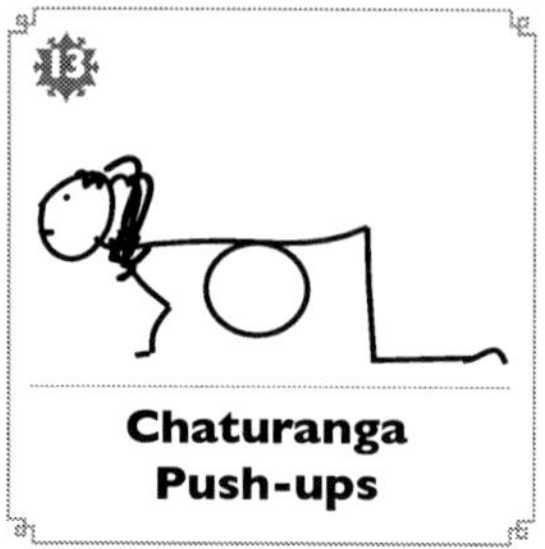

Chaturanga Push-ups

3x. Knees on floor.

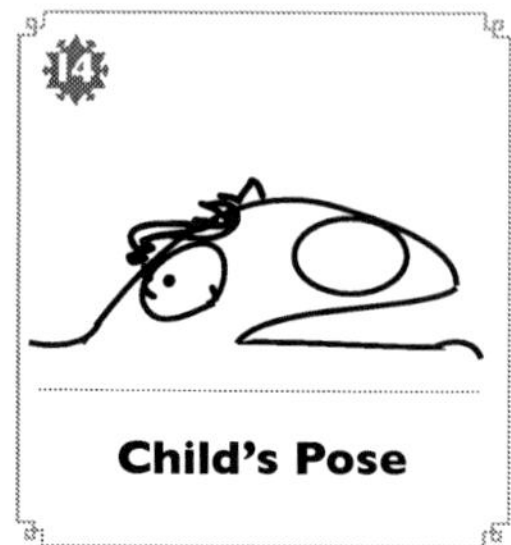

Child's Pose

Knees wide, toes together, arms forward.

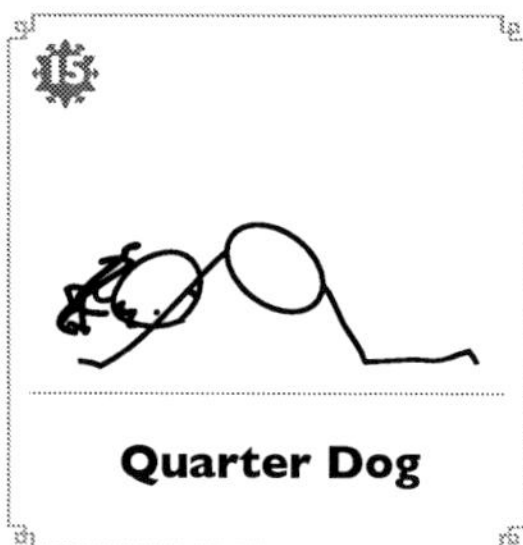

Quarter Dog

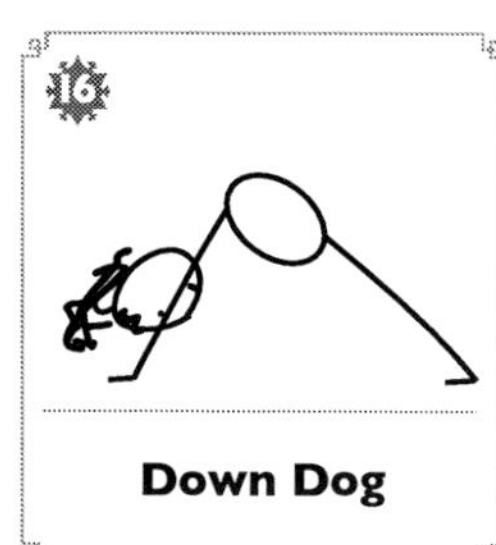

Down Dog

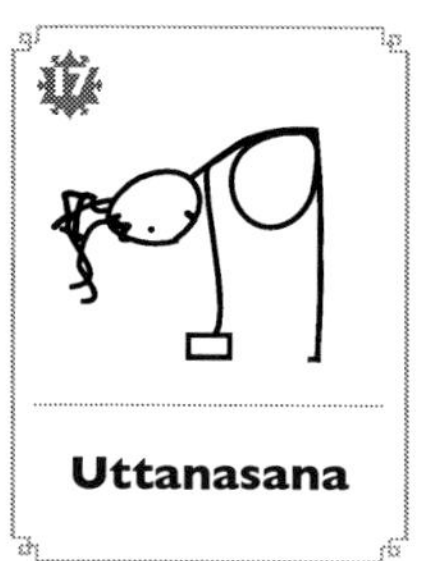

Uttanasana

Bend knees, hands on thighs to stand.

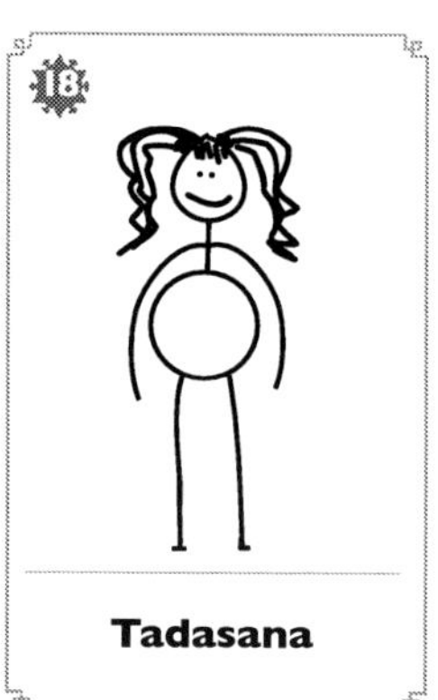

Tadasana

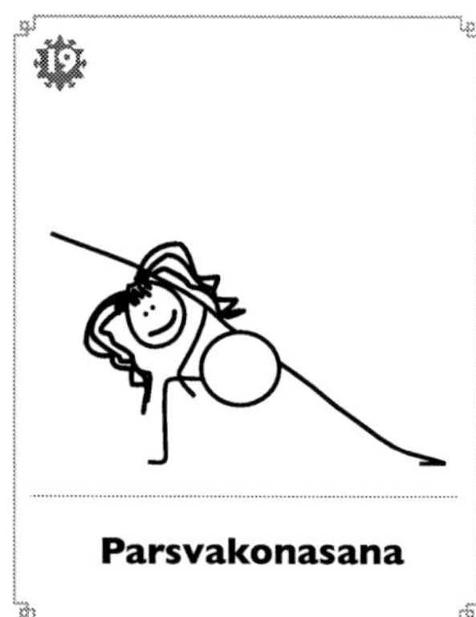

Parsvakonasana

Forearm to thigh or hand to block. Both sides.

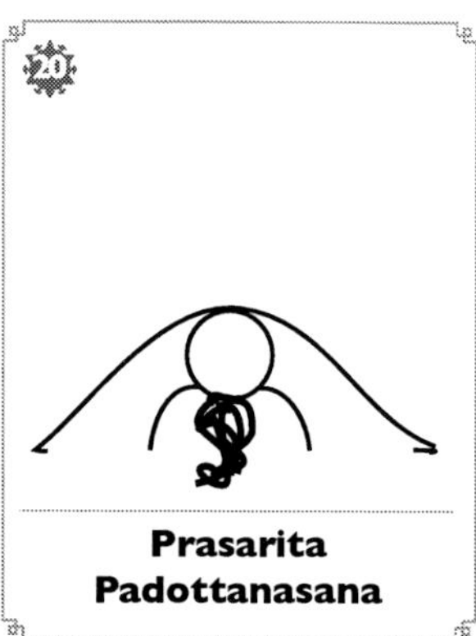

Prasarita Padottanasana

With block under hands if needed. Fold down the middle.

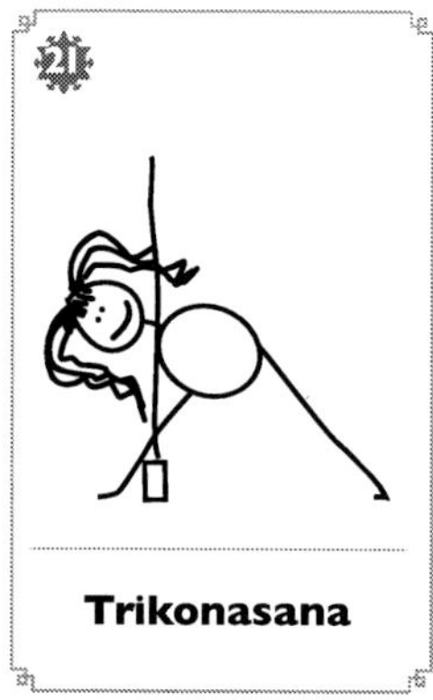

Trikonasana

With block if needed. Both sides.

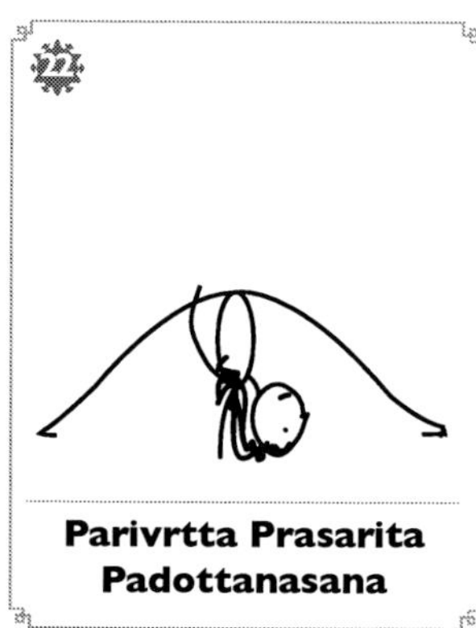

Parivrtta Prasarita Padottanasana

With gentle open-belly twist.

...continued on next page

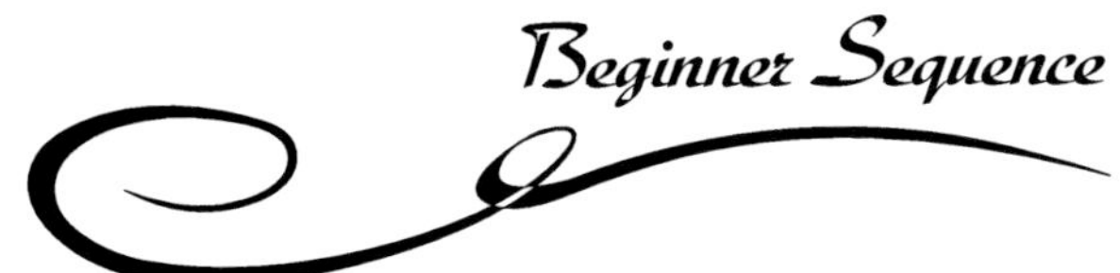

Beginner Sequence

...continued from page 92

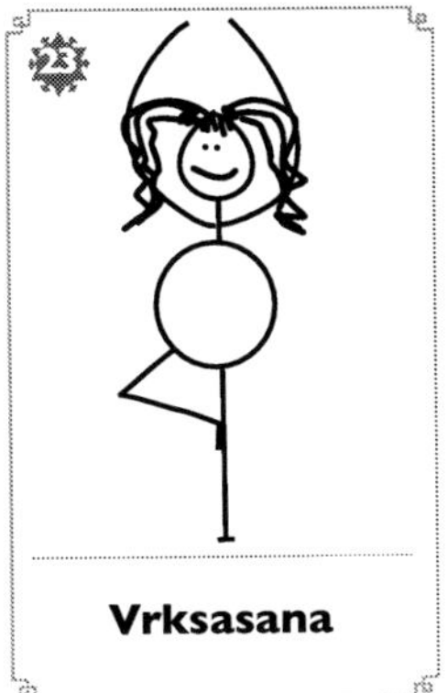

Vrksasana

With wall behind back.

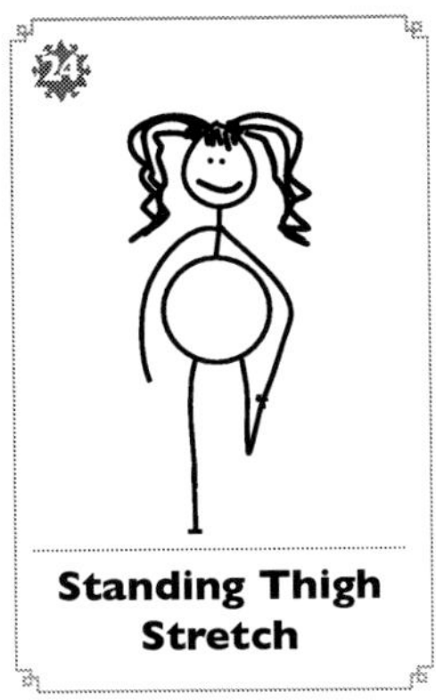

Standing Thigh Stretch

Hold wall if needed, breathe into back body.

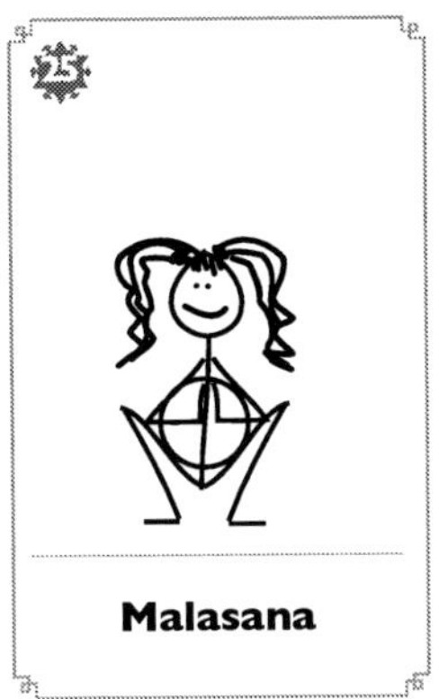

Malasana

At wall, practice kegels, use block under sitting bones if necessary.

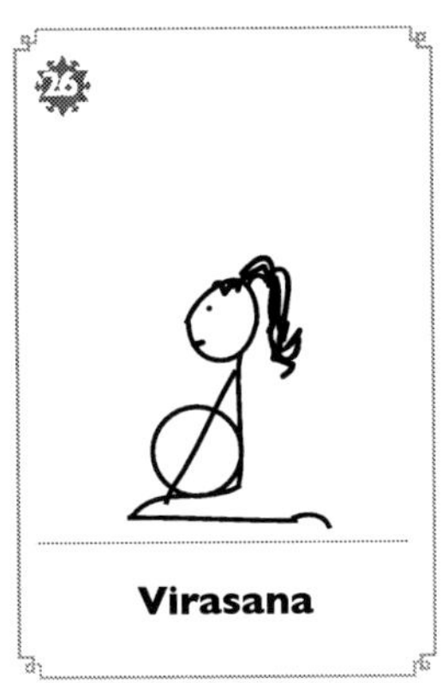

Virasana

Use block or blanket if needed.

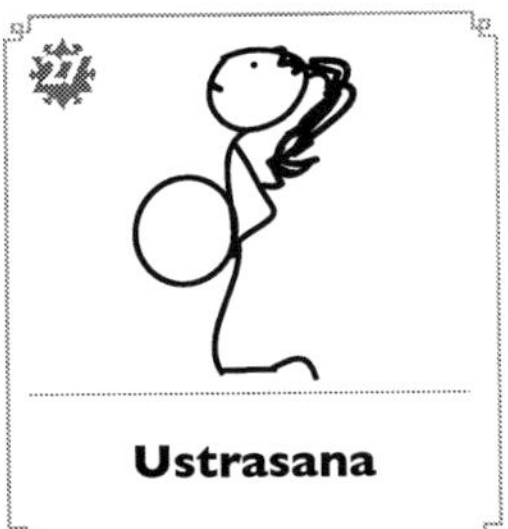

Ustrasana

With slight upper backbend, keep hands on hips.

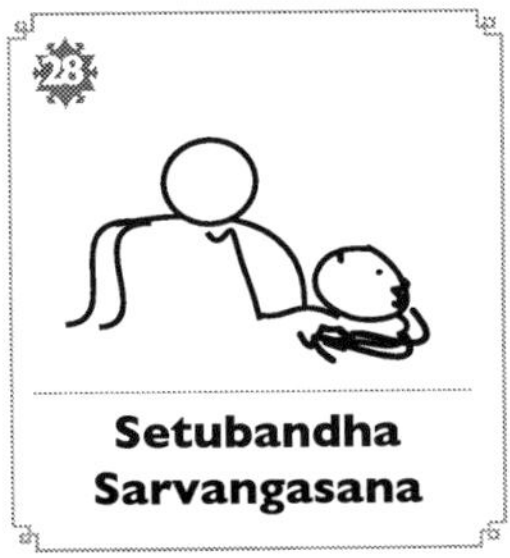

Setubandha Sarvangasana

Gentle lift of hips if comfortable. 3x. Rest on left side in between.

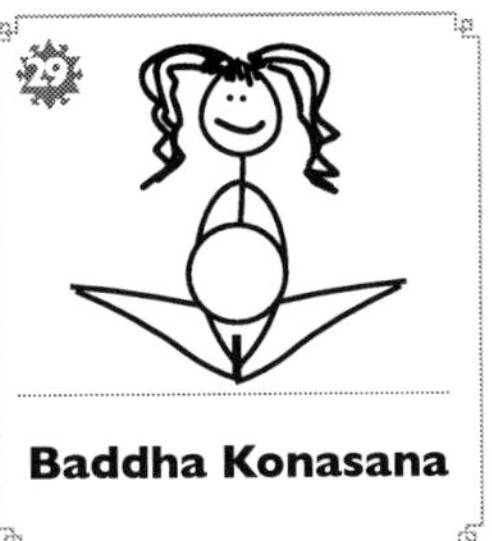

Baddha Konasana

Feet apart to fold forward.

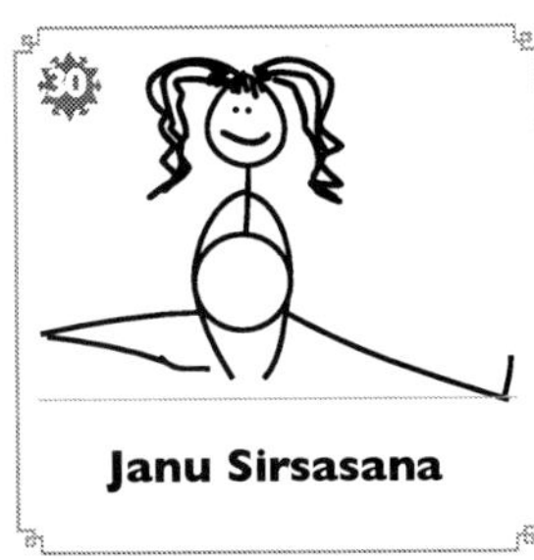

Janu Sirsasana

Fold between the legs.

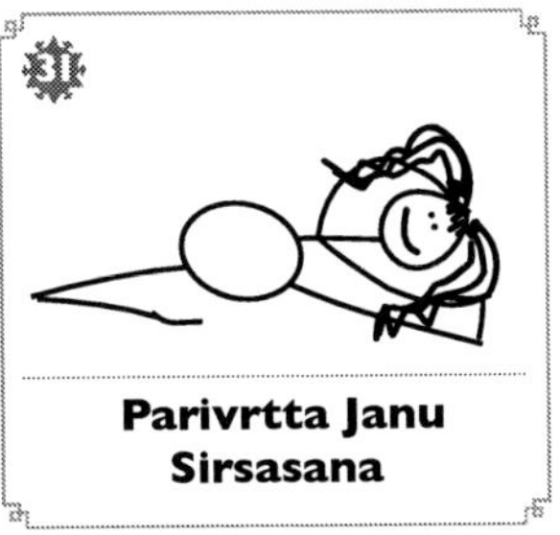

Parivrtta Janu Sirsasana

Place the top hand behind the base of the skull and the bottom hand on the floor.

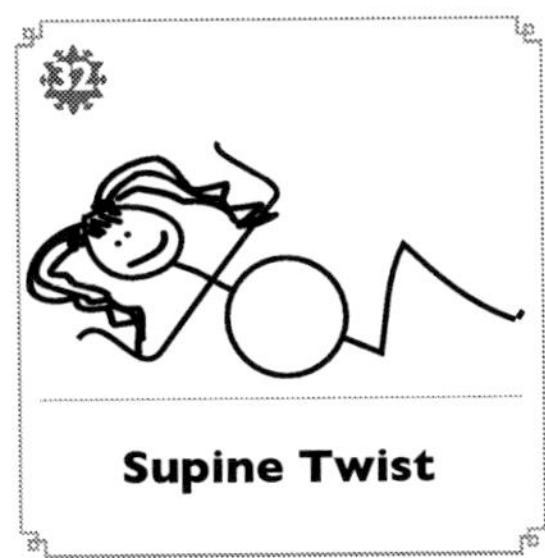

Supine Twist

Knees bent away from belly.

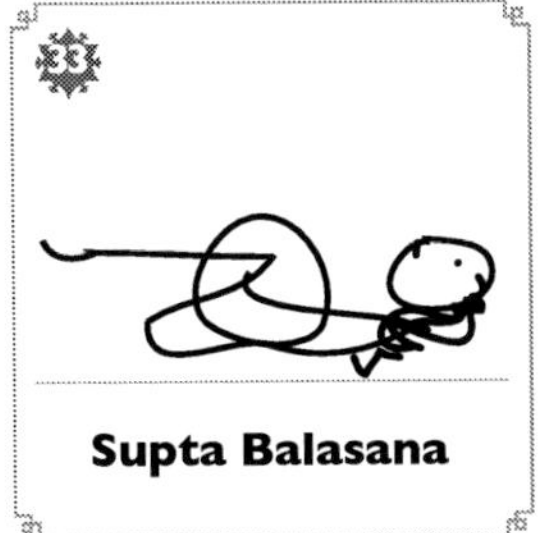

Supta Balasana

Lift head above heart after 4th month.

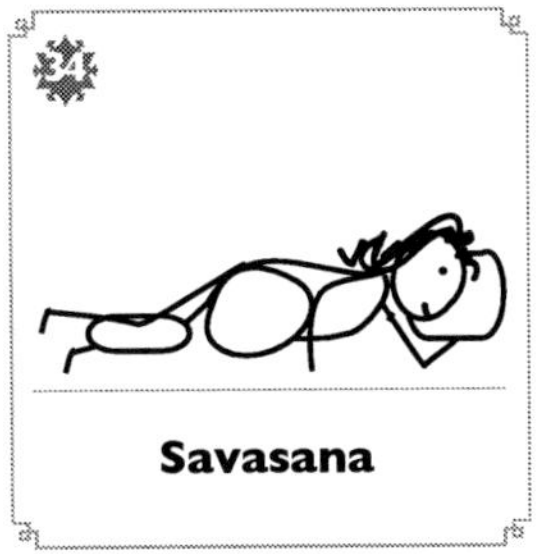

Savasana

With props on left side and between legs.

Wall Sequence (Mixed Level)

The wall is one of the most useful prenatal 'props' — it ensures stability and increases one's ability to engage and open the body. This sequence can be modified according to the level of the practitioner, and poses can be eliminated to shorten the length of the sequence.

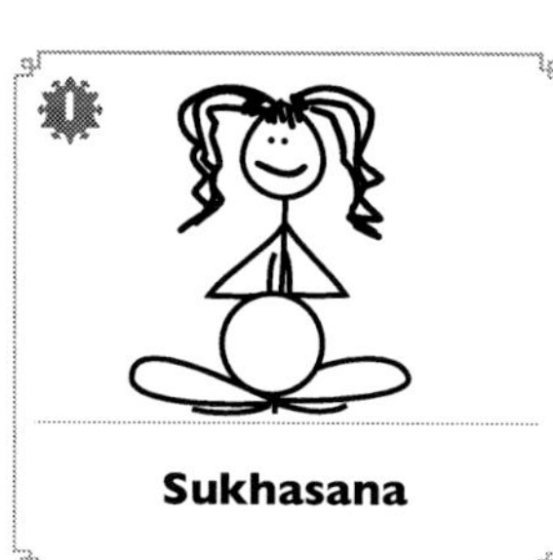

Sukhasana

On blanket for opening meditation.

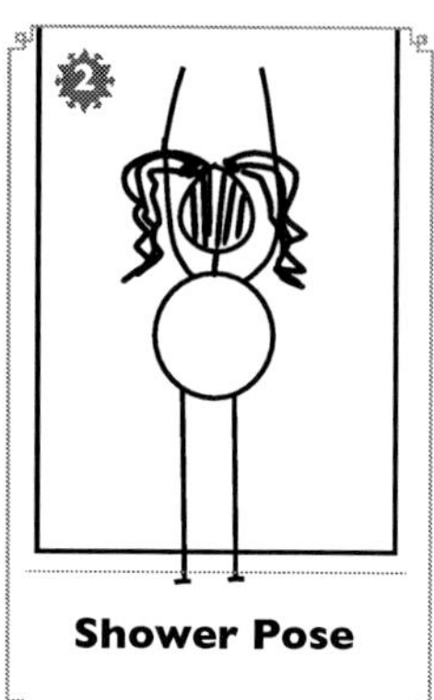

Shower Pose

Standing facing the wall (2 feet away), arms overhead, hands at wall.

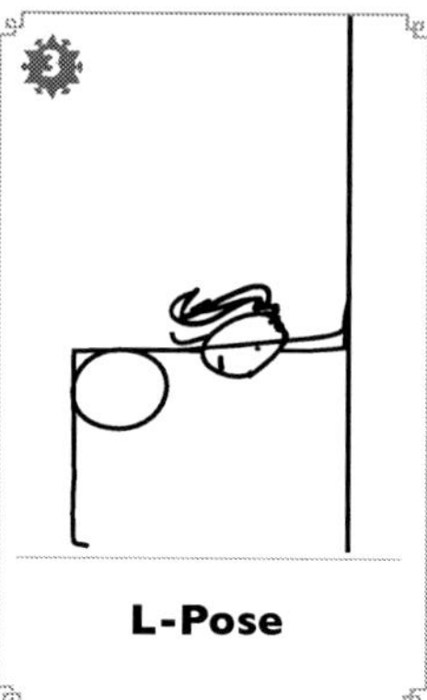

L-Pose

Torso parallel to floor, hips over heels.

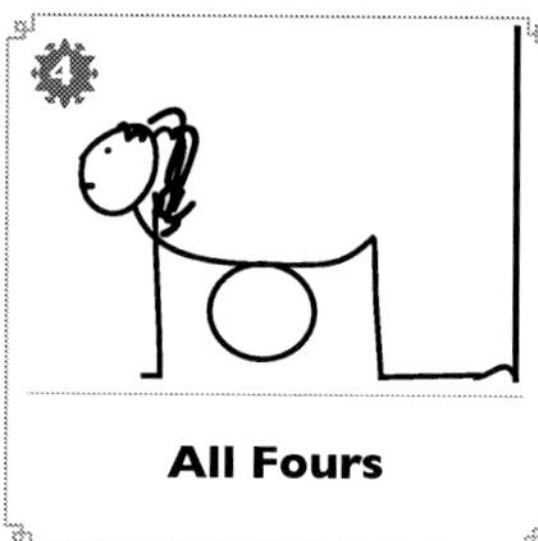

All Fours

Facing away from wall. Root hands, strengthen arms, soften heart.

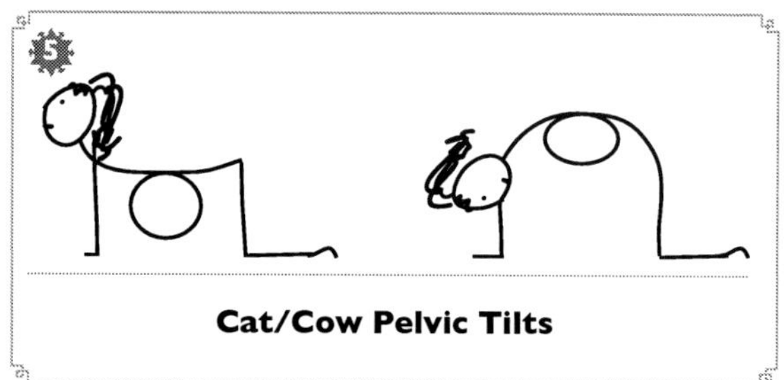

Cat/Cow Pelvic Tilts

5x. Link breath with movement.

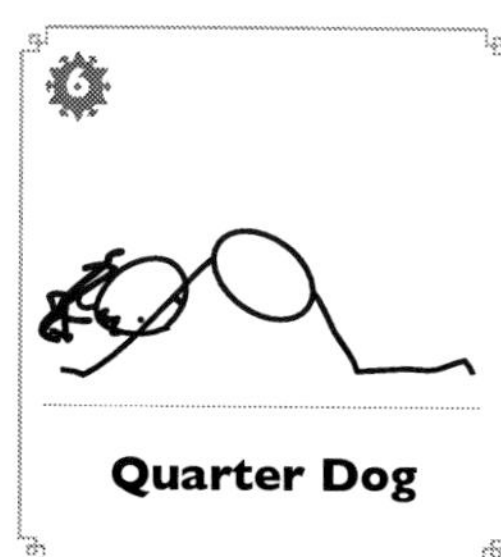

Quarter Dog

Knees on floor, arms angled back, arm bones lift.

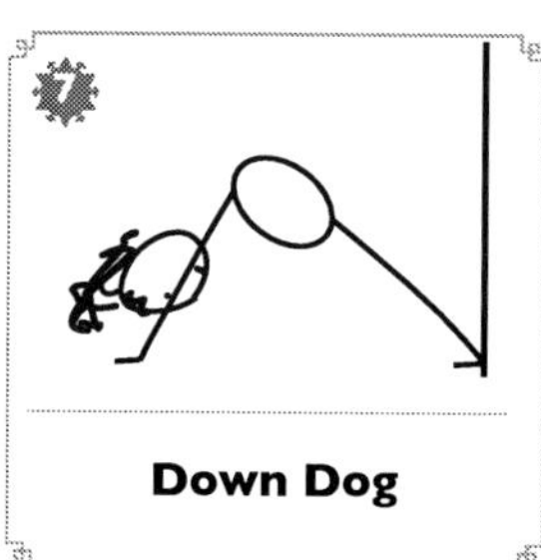

Down Dog

Heels up wall.

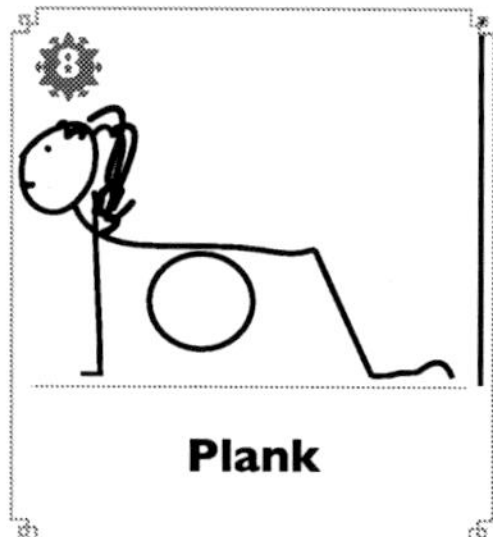

Plank

With knees on floor behind hips.

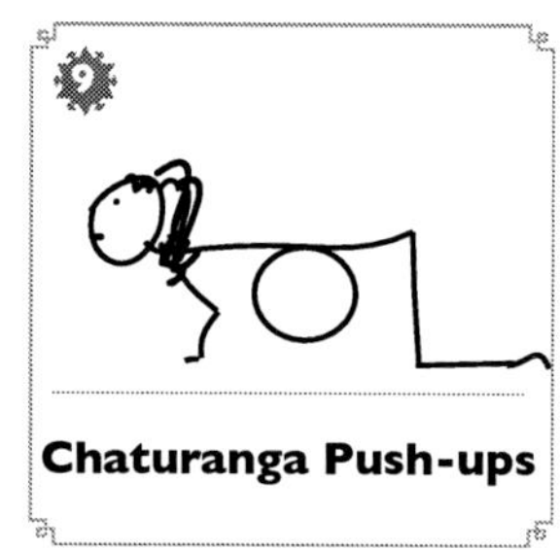

Chaturanga Push-ups

3x. Knees on floor.

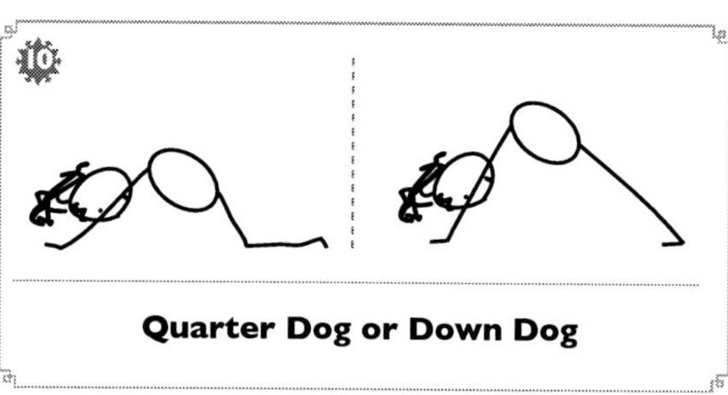

Quarter Dog or Down Dog

Then walk hands back to feet.

...continued on next page

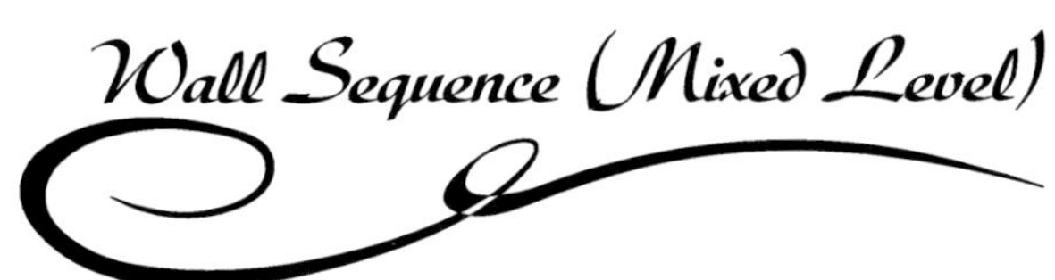

Wall Sequence (Mixed Level)

...continued from page 94

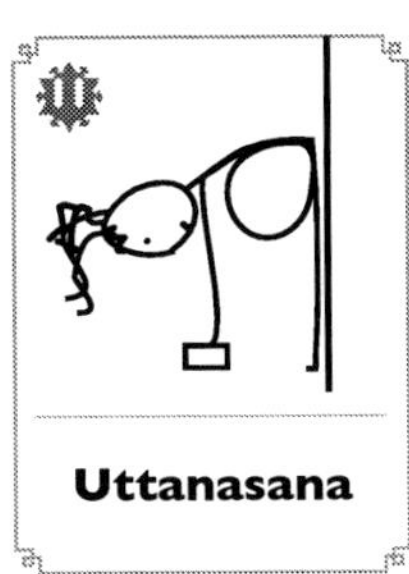

Uttanasana

With hands elevated on blocks if needed. Thighs back towards wall.

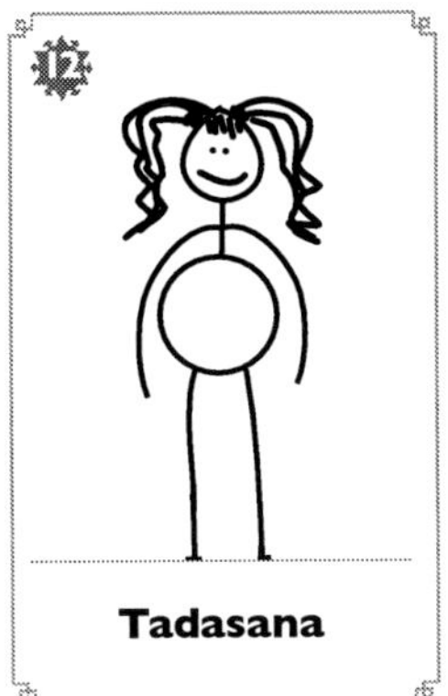

Tadasana

Step slightly away from wall.

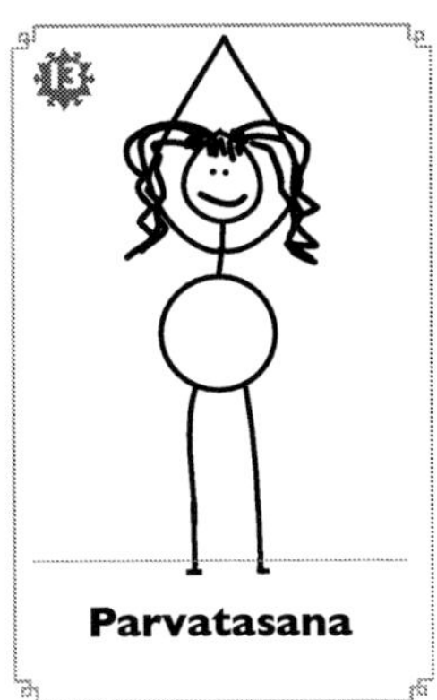

Parvatasana

Arms overhead, lift heels (use wall for balance).

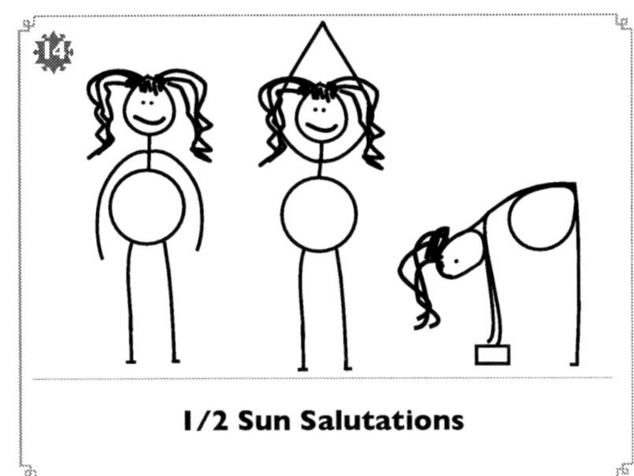

1/2 Sun Salutations

3x. Hands on blocks if needed.

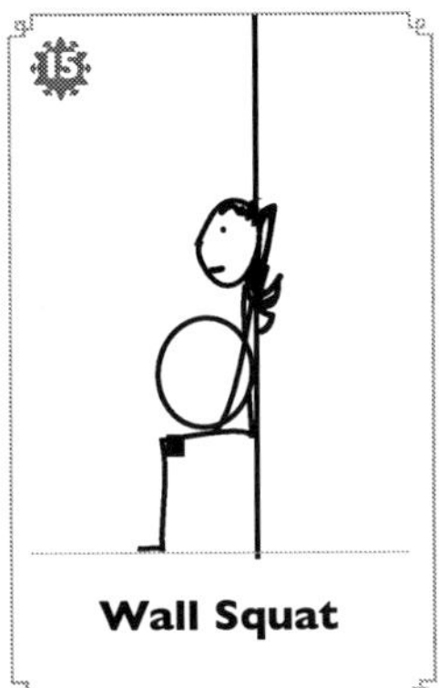

Wall Squat

1 minute. 2x. Lean against wall with block between legs.

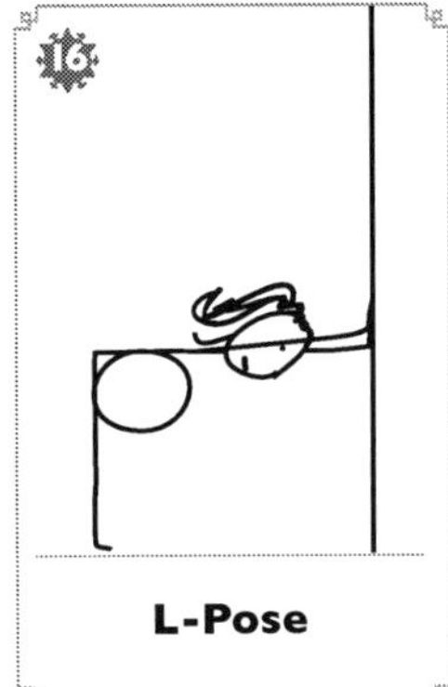

L-Pose

From L-pose, move left foot to wall for standing pose.

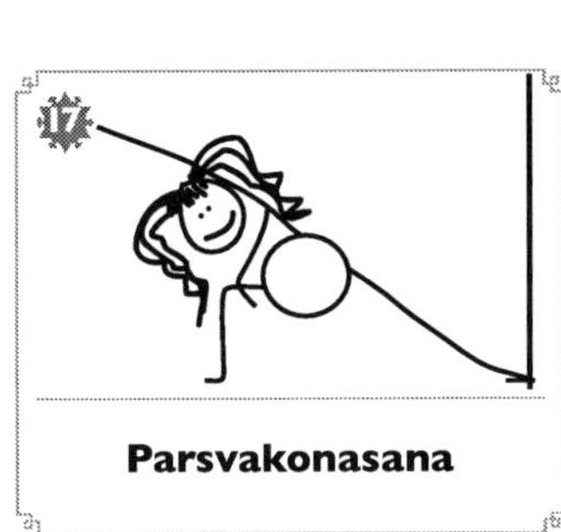

Parsvakonasana

Forearm to thigh or hand to block (back foot pressing against wall).

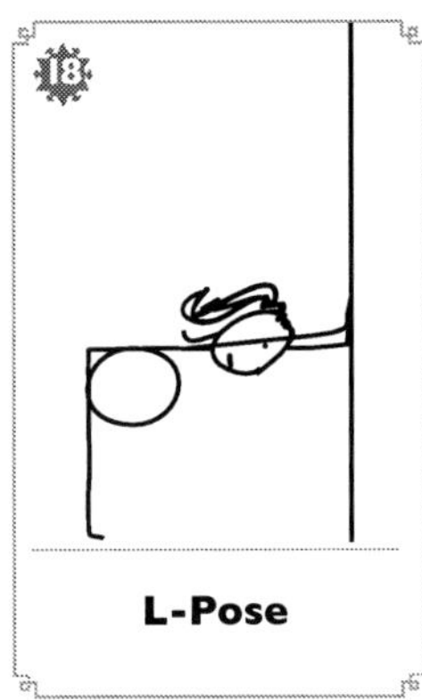

L-Pose

L-pose in between right and left side.

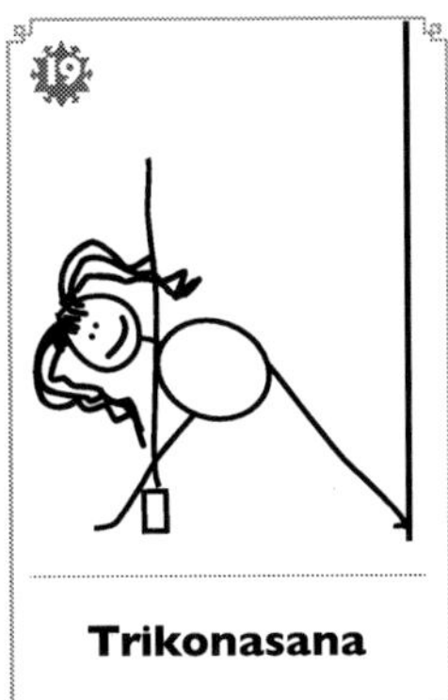

Trikonasana

Use block if needed (back foot pressing against wall).

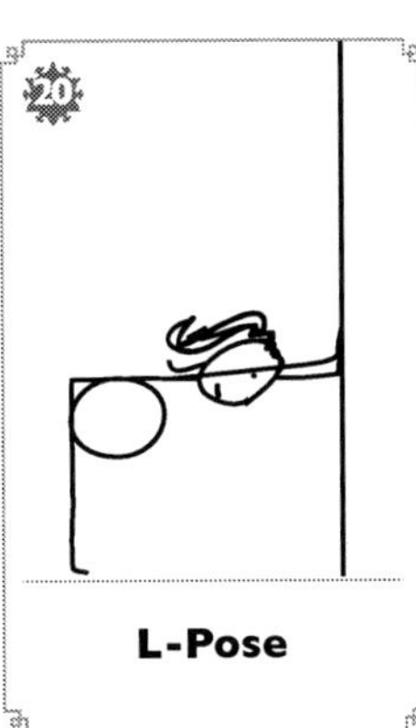

L-Pose

L-pose in between right and left side.

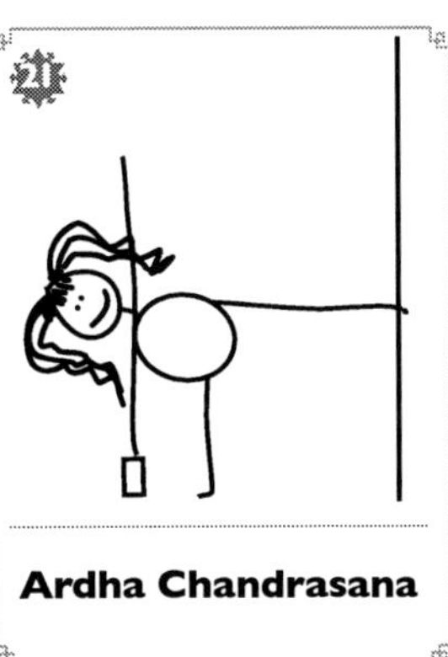

Ardha Chandrasana

With foot on wall or leaning against wall. Use block if needed.

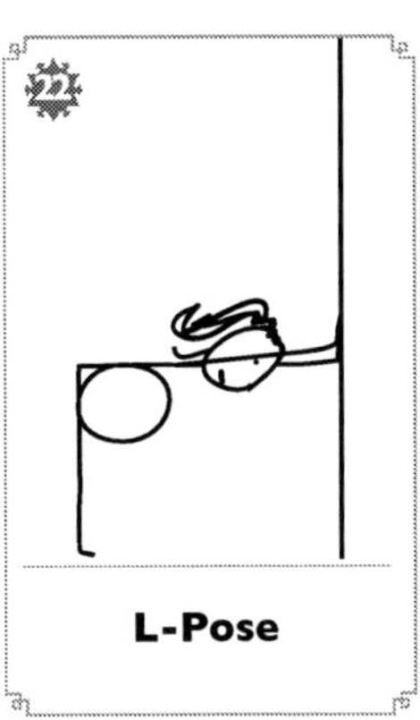

L-Pose

L-pose in between right and left side.

...continued on next page

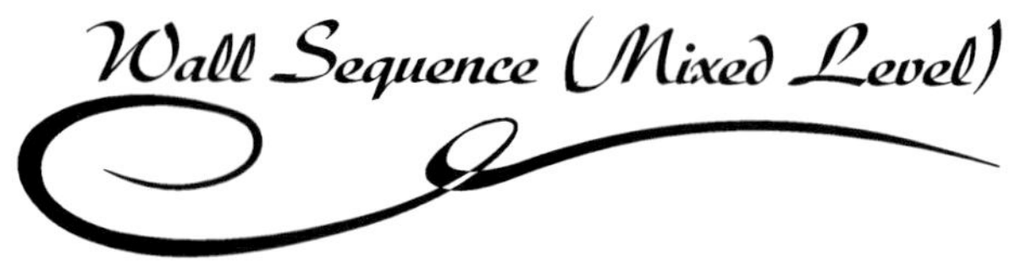

Wall Sequence (Mixed Level)

...continued from page 95

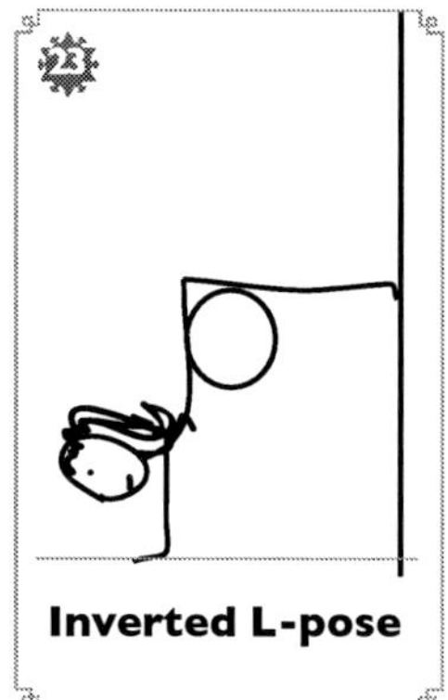

Inverted L-pose

(1/2 handstands) if comfortable.

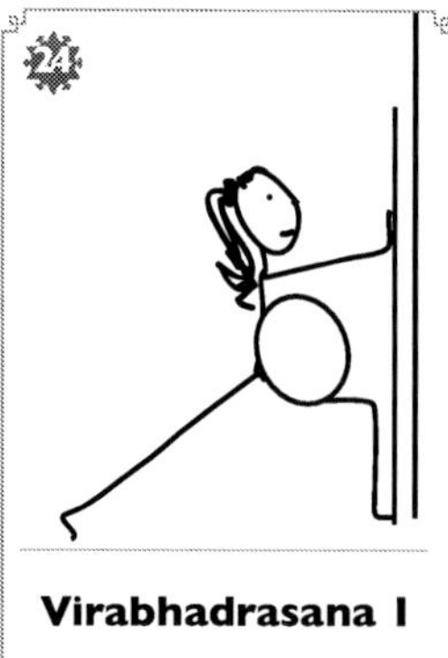

Virabhadrasana 1

Facing wall with back heel up – straighten and bend front leg with breath.

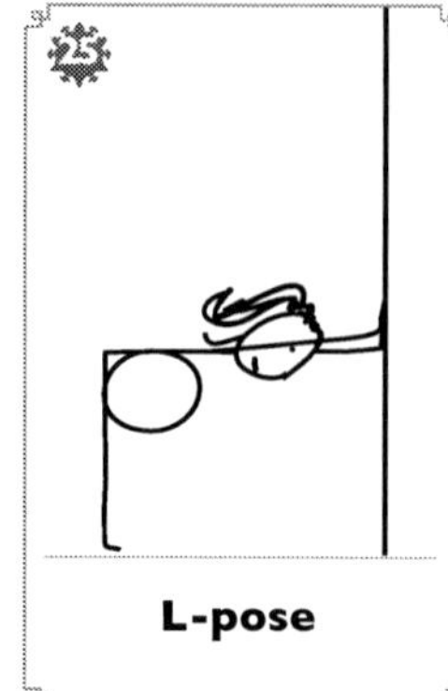

L-pose

Torso parallel to floor, hips over heels.

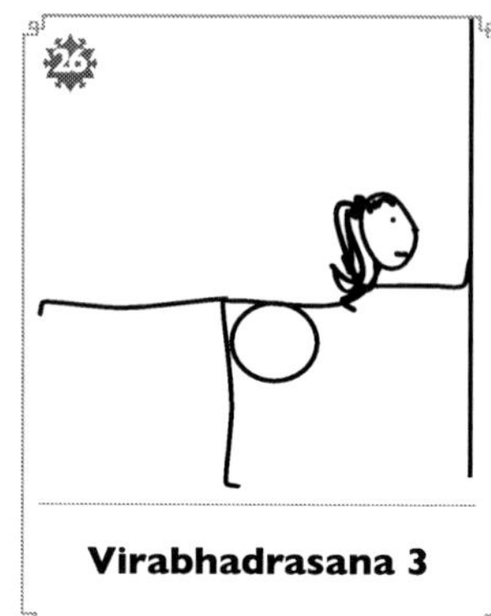

Virabhadrasana 3

With hands at wall, leg lower than hip.

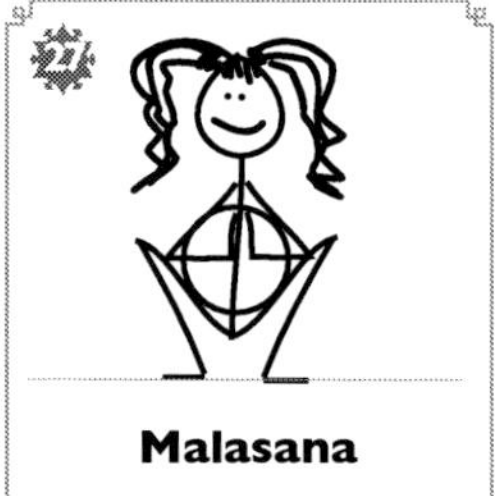

Malasana

At wall – practice kegels.

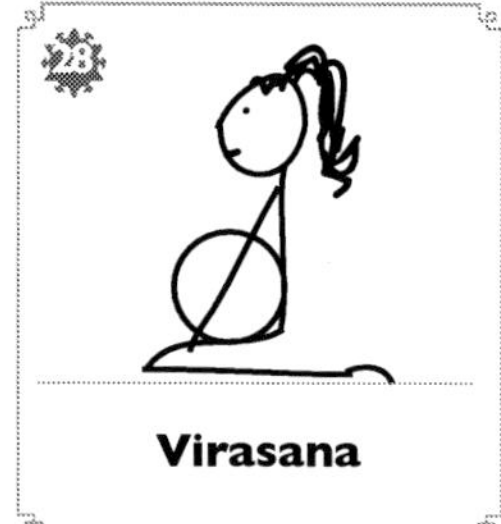

Virasana

Then with slight upper backbend (or supta with block behind back, first trimester only).

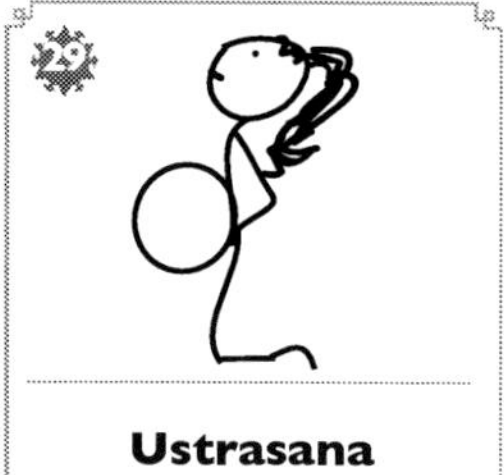

Ustrasana

With slight upper backbend or hands to heels (if comfortable).

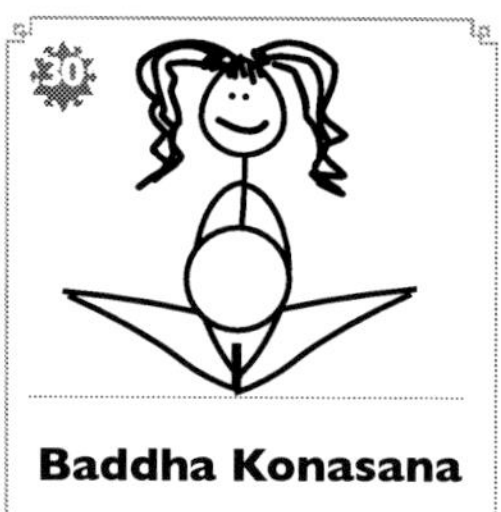

Baddha Konasana

Feet apart to fold forward.

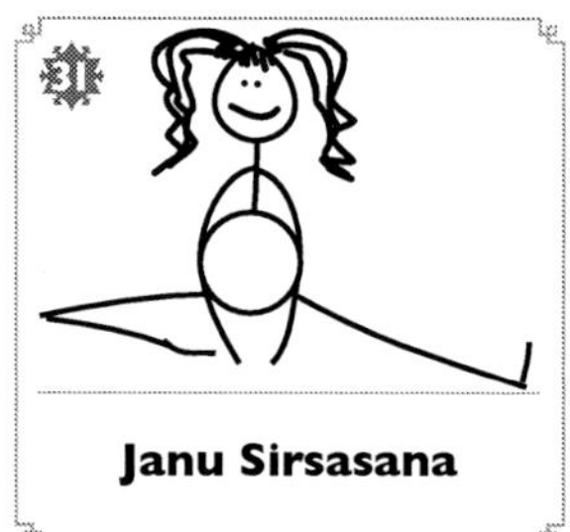

Janu Sirsasana

Fold between legs.

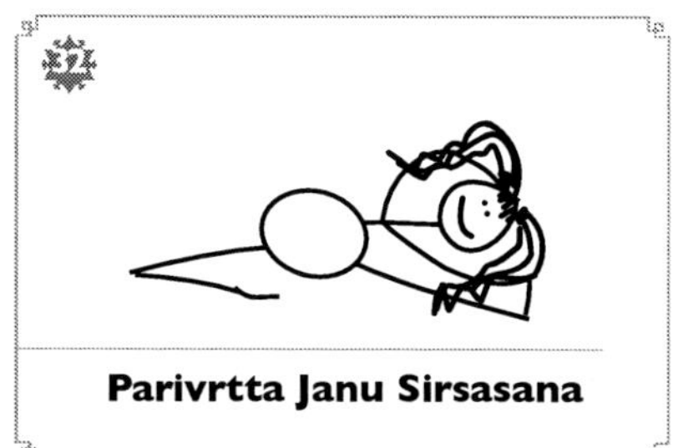

Parivrtta Janu Sirsasana

Place the top hand behind the base of the skull and the bottom hand on the floor.

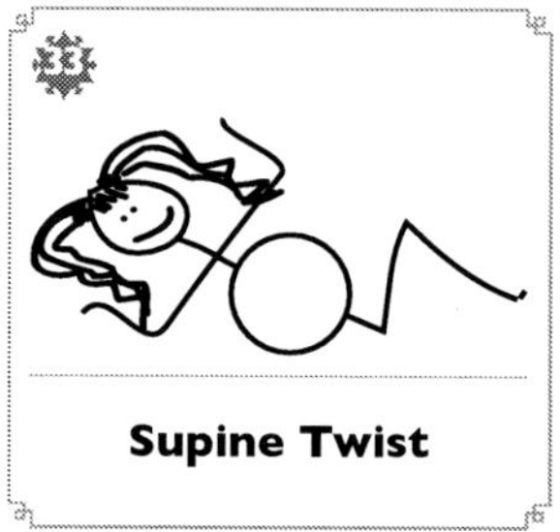

Supine Twist

Knees bent away from belly.

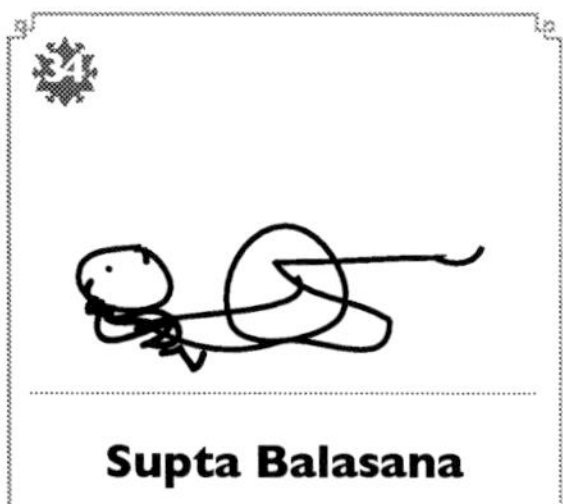

Supta Balasana

Lift head above heart after 4th month.

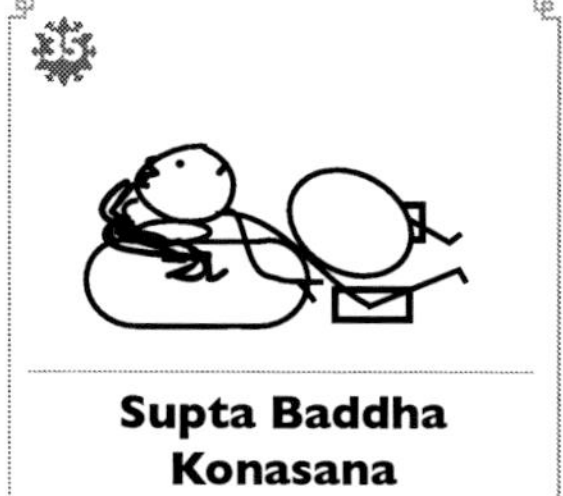

Supta Baddha Konasana

With blocks under knees and bolster under torso.

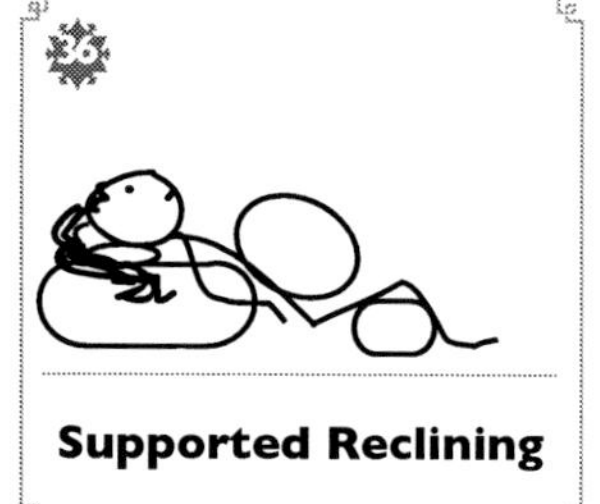

Supported Reclining

With bolster under torso and knees.

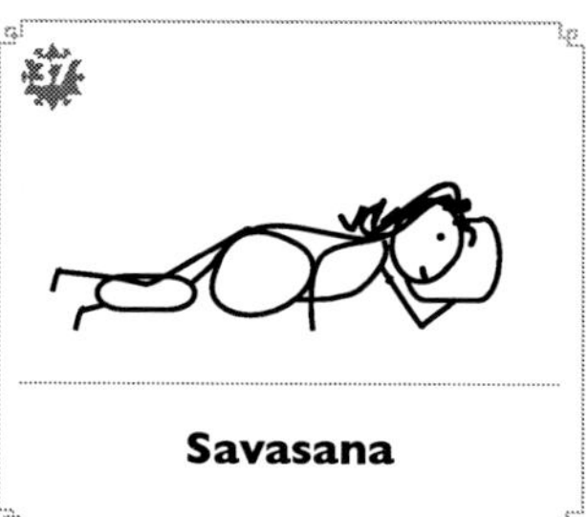

Savasana

With props on left side and between legs.

Intermediate Sequence

This practice is for experienced yoginis comfortable in these poses before getting pregnant. It is advisable to work slowly to decide each day whether to modify or leave out poses.

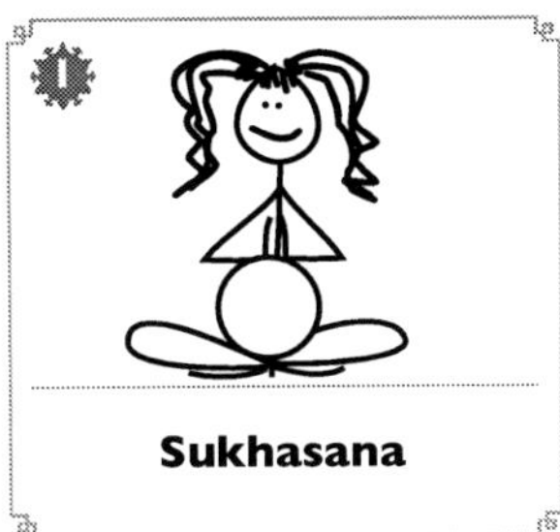

Sukhasana

On blanket for opening meditation.

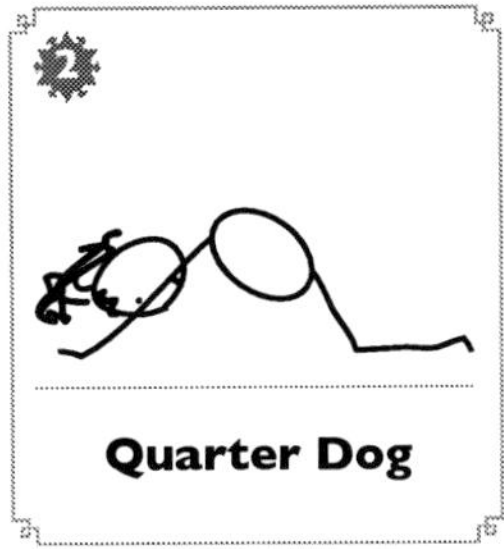

Quarter Dog

Knees on floor, arms angled back, arm bones lift.

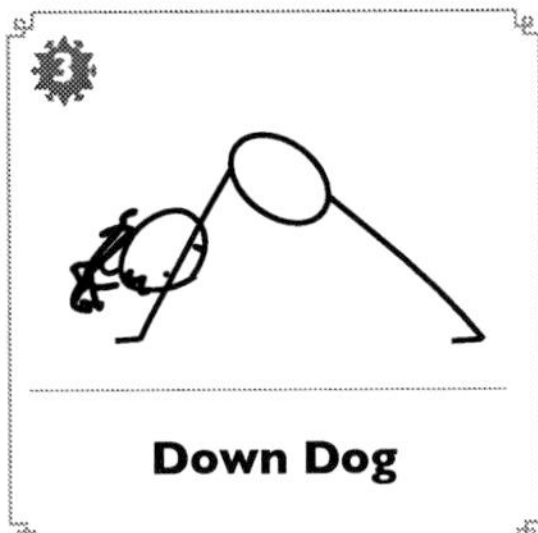

Down Dog

Wide legs, walk feet out. Then, walk hands back to feet.

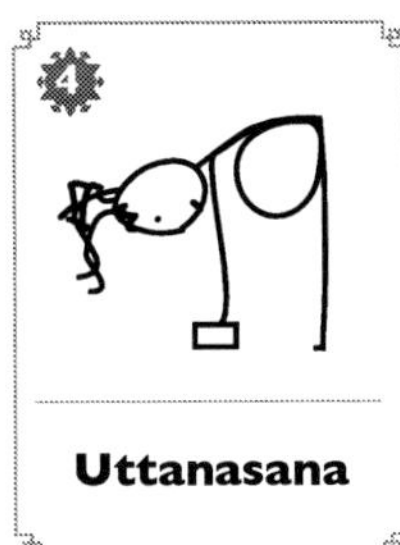

Uttanasana

With hands elevated on blocks if needed.

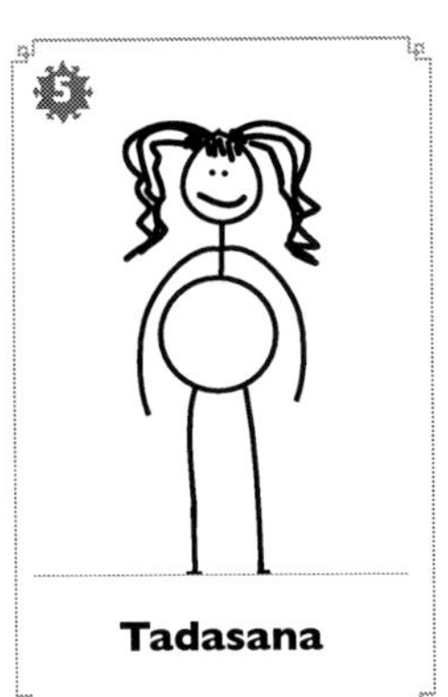

Tadasana

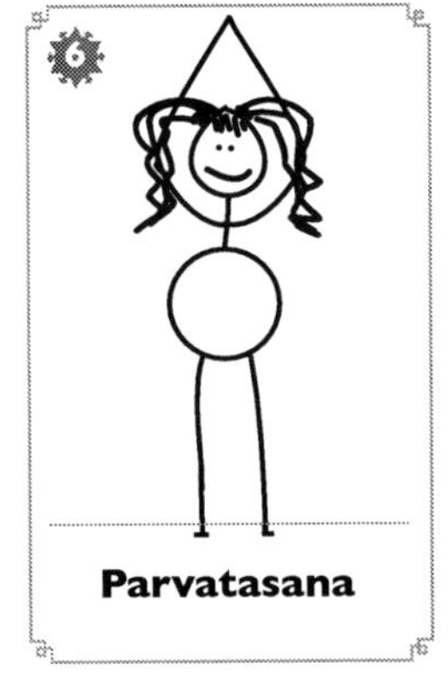

Parvatasana

Arms overhead, then arms clasped behind back.

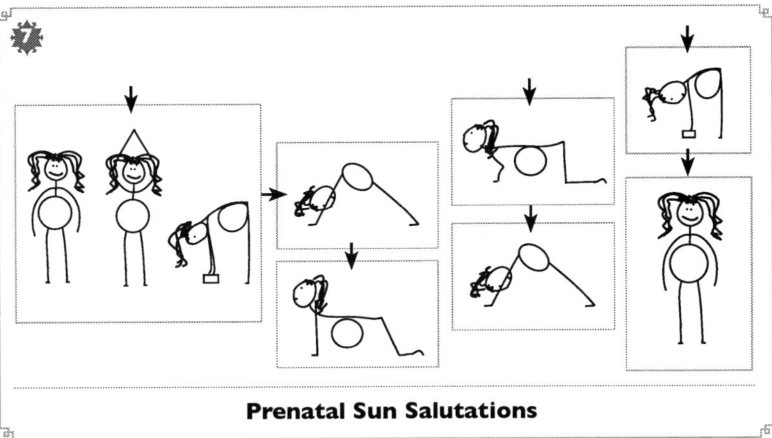

Prenatal Sun Salutations

3x. Walk forward into Down Dog, Plank with knees on floor, Chaturanga, Cobra (if it feels ok), Down Dog, walk hands to feet for Uttanasana, Tadasana.

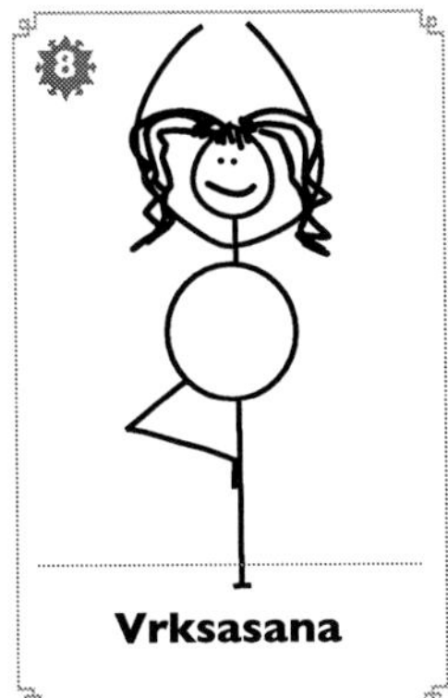

Vrksasana

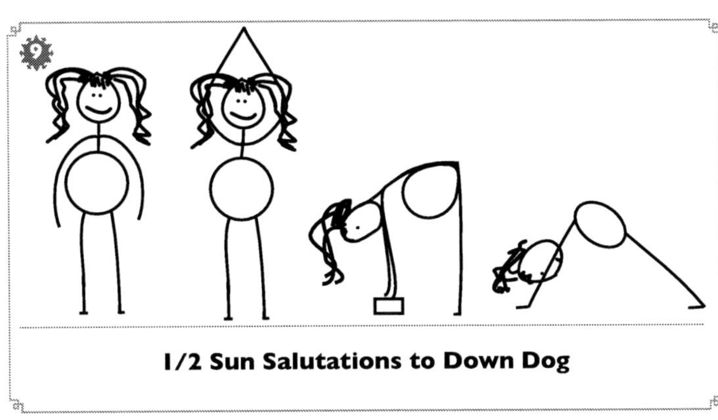

1/2 Sun Salutations to Down Dog

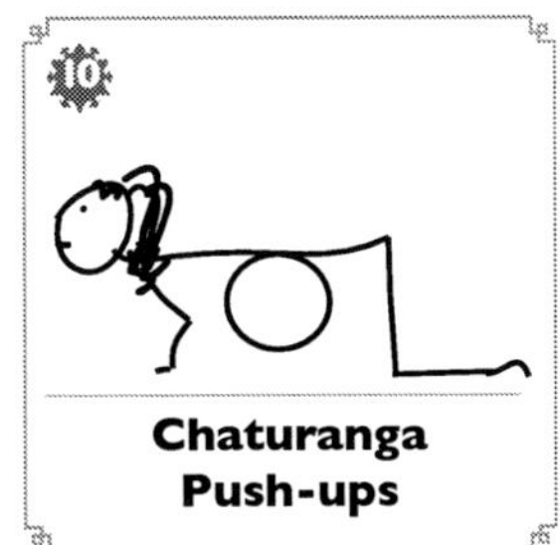

Chaturanga Push-ups

3x. Knees on floor. Lift heels of hands if possible.

...continued on next page

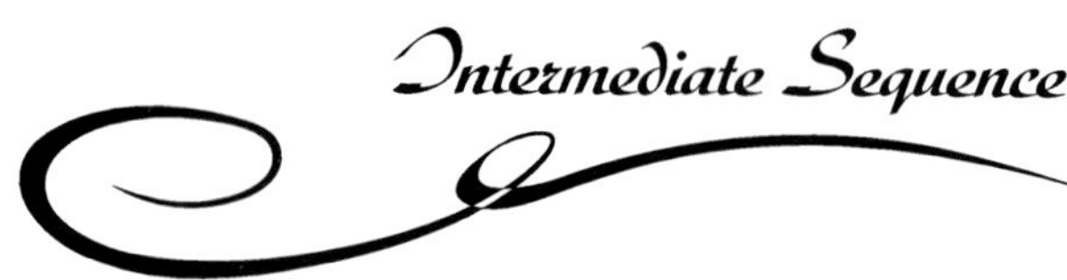

Intermediate Sequence

...continued from page 97

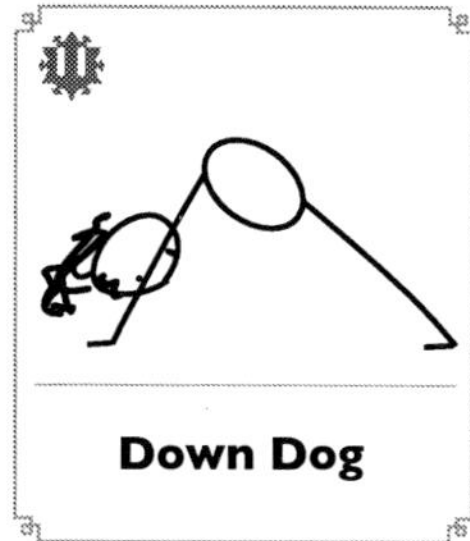

Down Dog

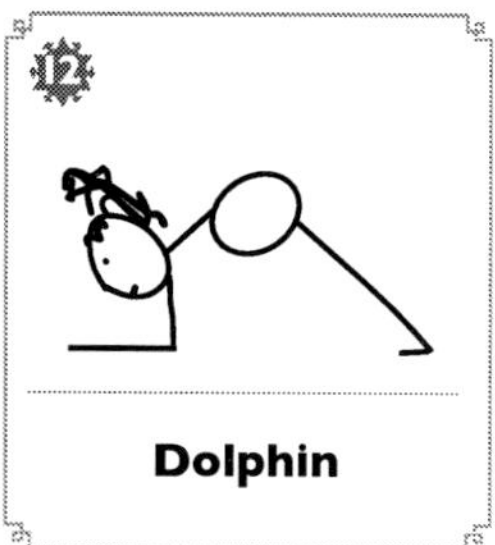

Dolphin

Forearms to floor. Then Down Dog, walk hands to feet.

Utkatasana

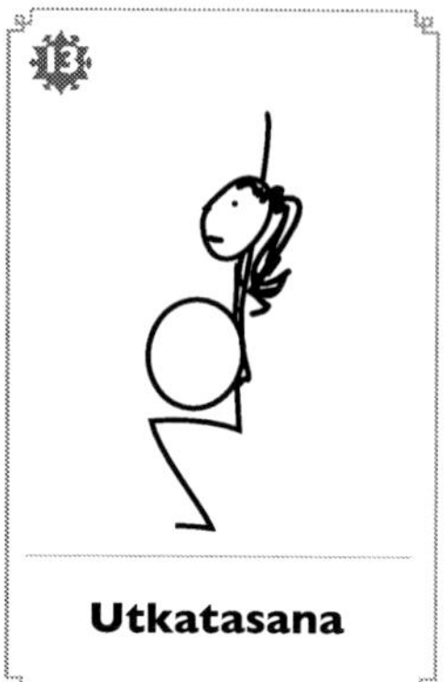

Parsvakonasana

Forearm to thigh or hand to block. Both sides.

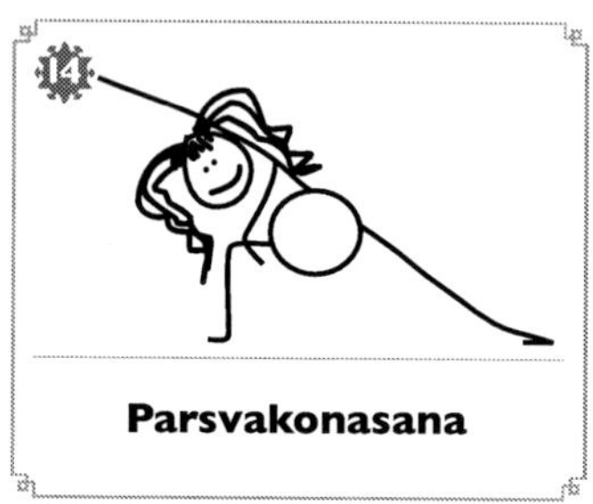

Prasarita Padottanasana

Fold down the middle.

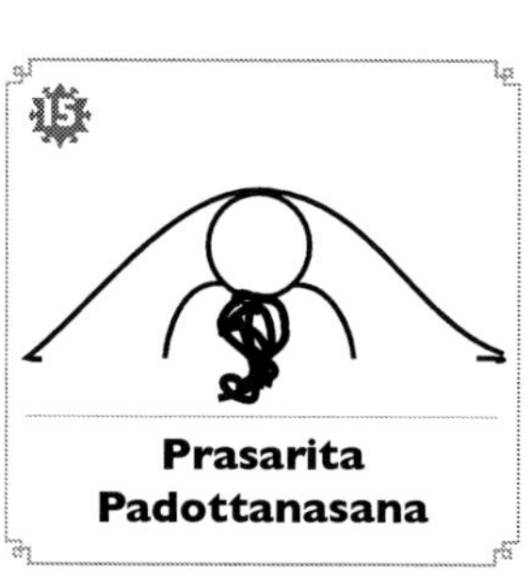

Trikonasana

With block if needed. Both sides.

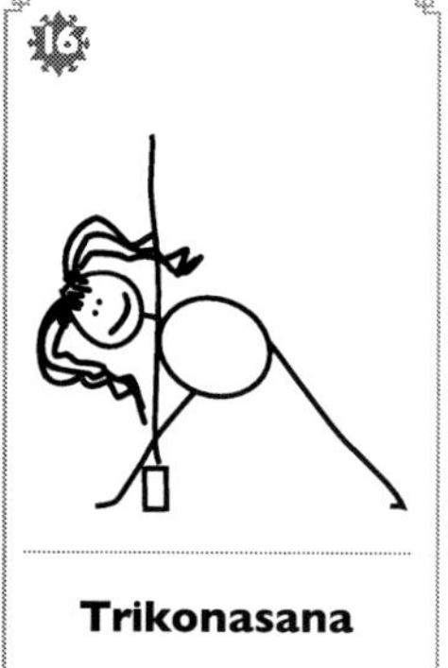

Parivrtta Prasarita Padottanasana

With gentle open-belly twist.

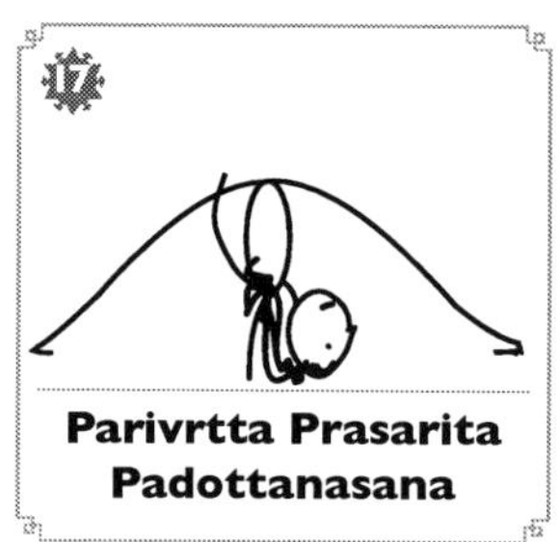

Ardha Chandrasana

With foot on wall or leaning against wall. Use block if needed.

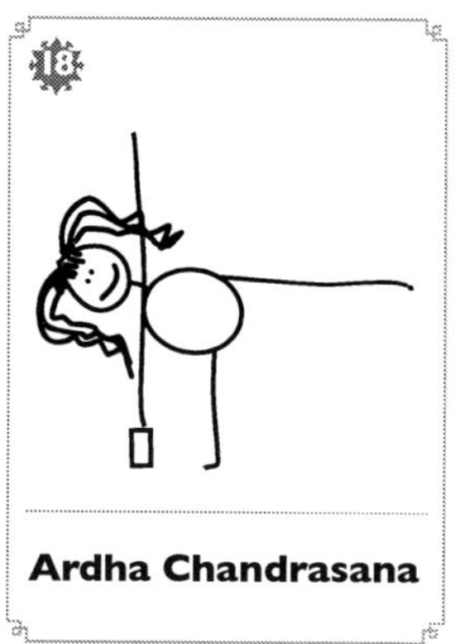

Handstands

Or 1/2 handstands at wall (if comfortable).

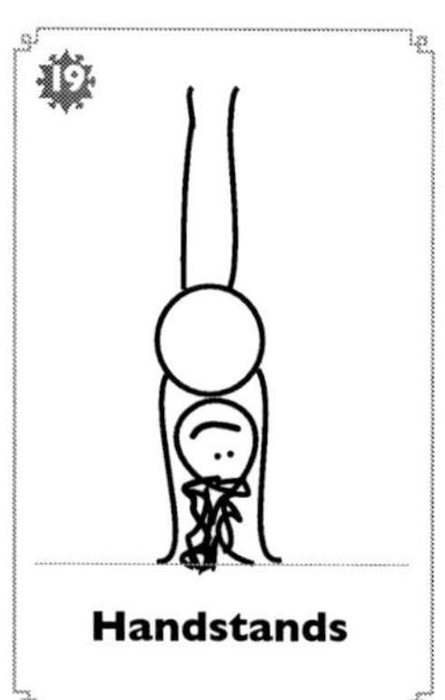

Virabhadrasana 3

Hands at wall, then let go.

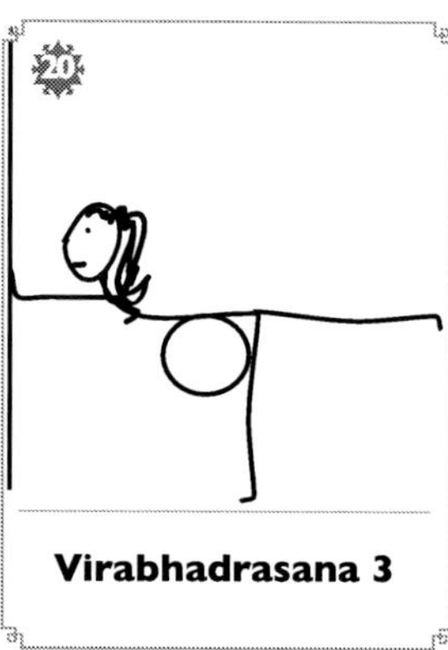

Wall Squat

1 minute. 2x. Lean against wall with block between legs.

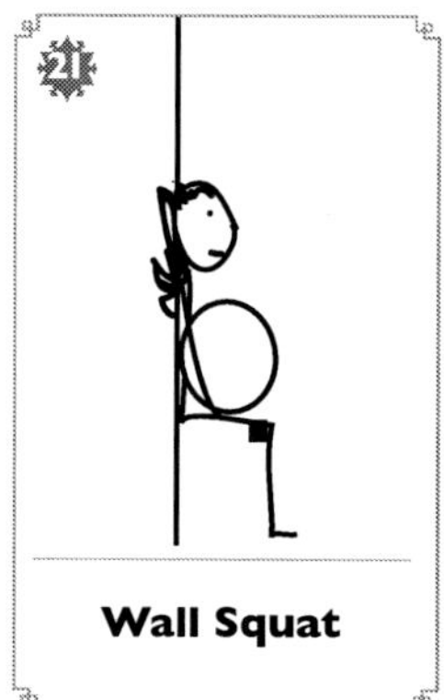

Standing Thigh Stretch

Hold wall if needed, breathe into back body.

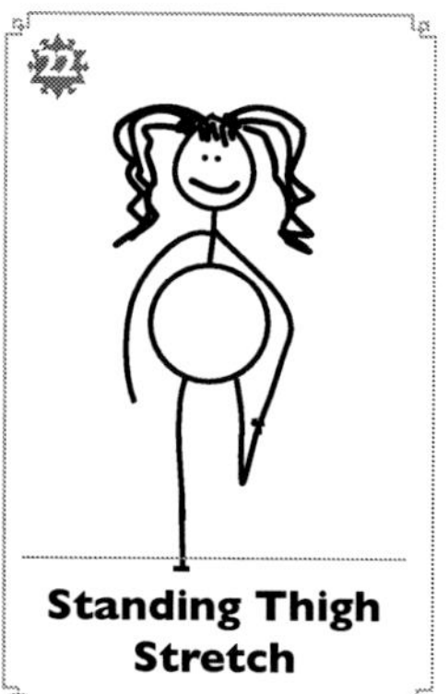

Malasana

Practice kegels.

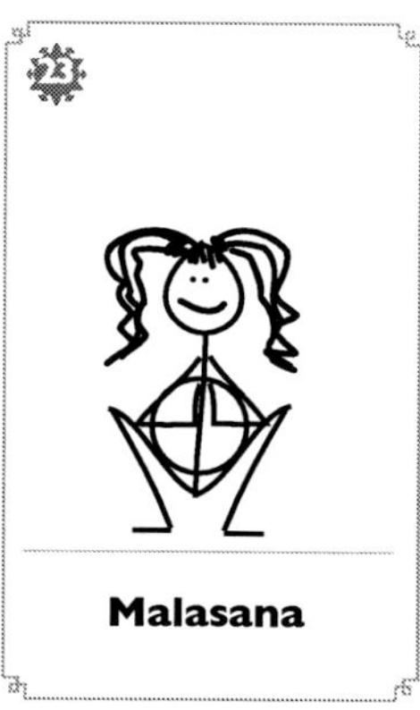

...continued on next page

...continued from page 98

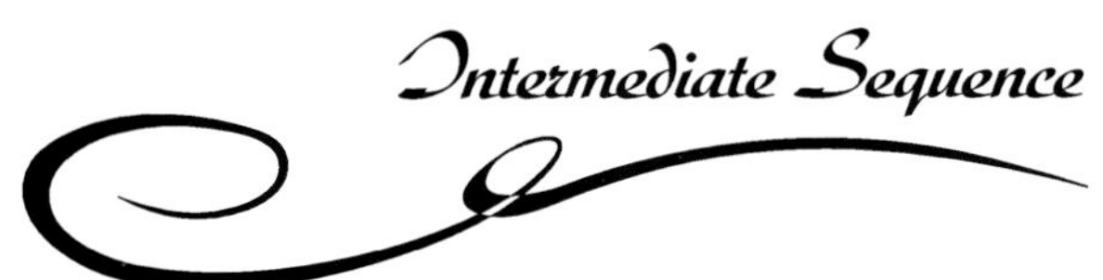

Intermediate Sequence

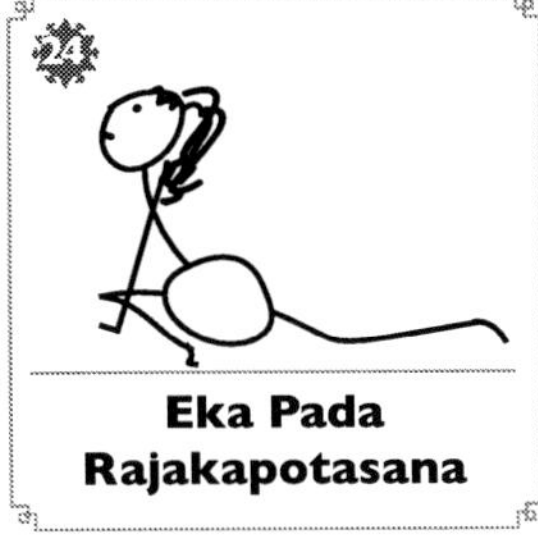

Eka Pada Rajakapotasana

Pigeon prep with legs fully engaged, torso upright.

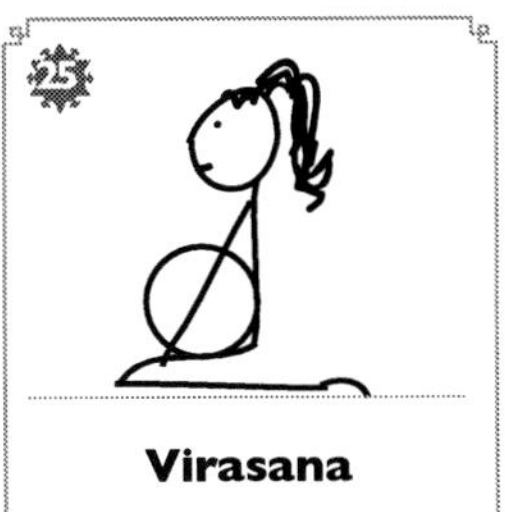

Virasana

Then with slight upper backbend (or supta with block behind back, first trimester only).

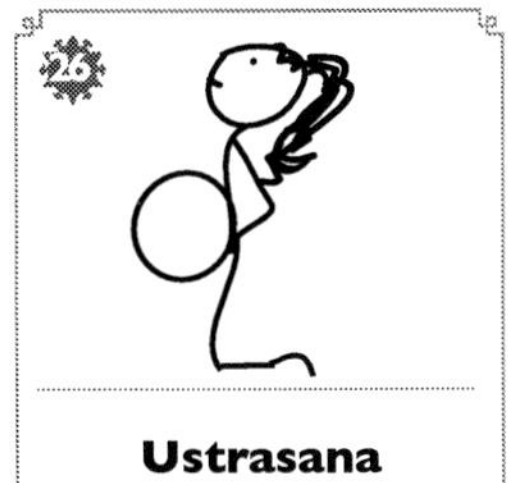

Ustrasana

With slight upper backbend or hands to heels (if comfortable).

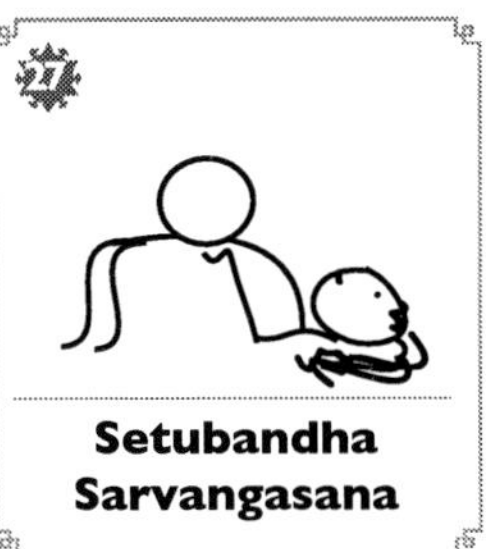

Setubandha Sarvangasana

Gentle lift of hips if comfortable. 3x. Rest on left side in between.

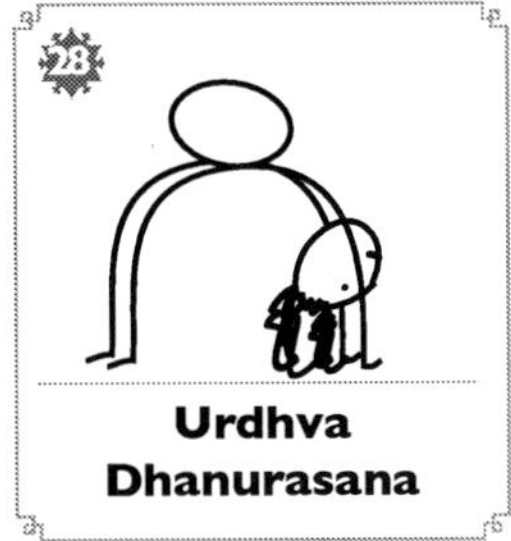

Urdhva Dhanurasana

If comfortable.

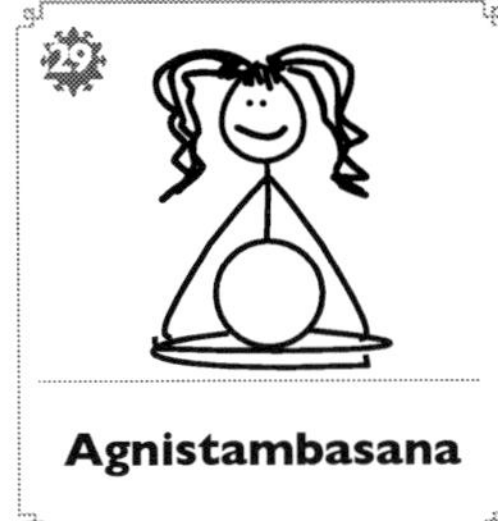

Agnistambasana

Keep feet active.

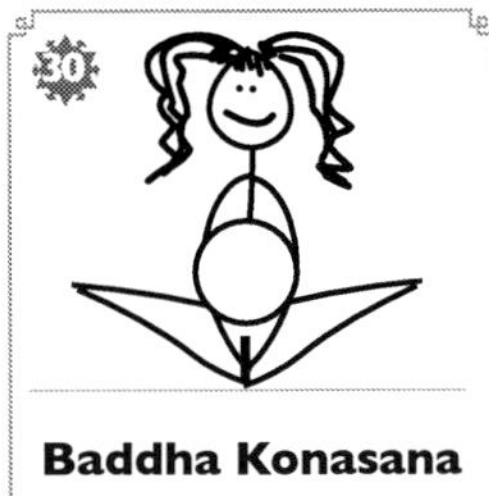

Baddha Konasana

Feet apart to fold forward.

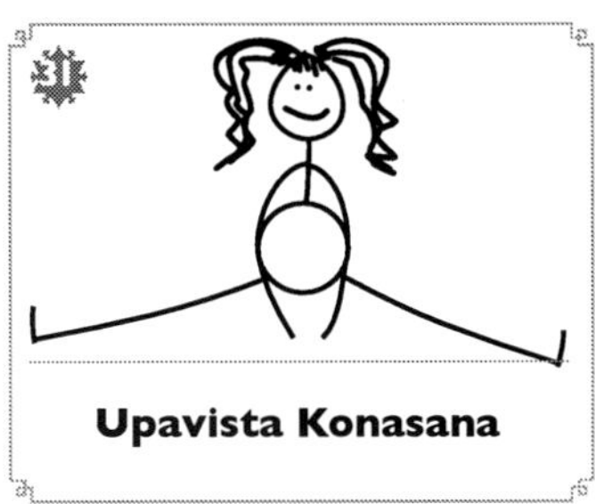

Upavista Konasana

Fold down middle.

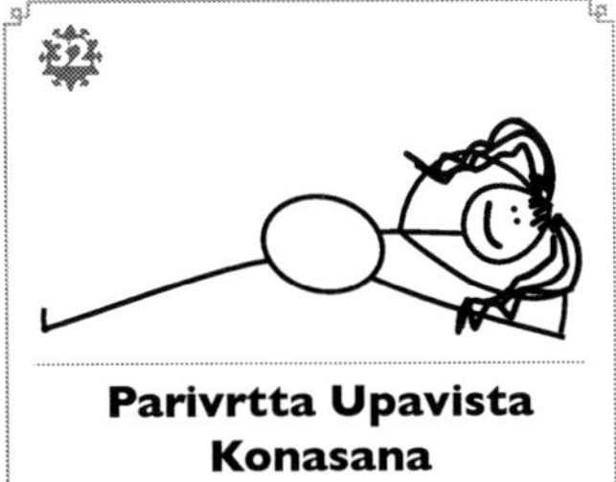

Parivrtta Upavista Konasana

Place the top hand behind the base of the skull and the bottom hand on the floor.

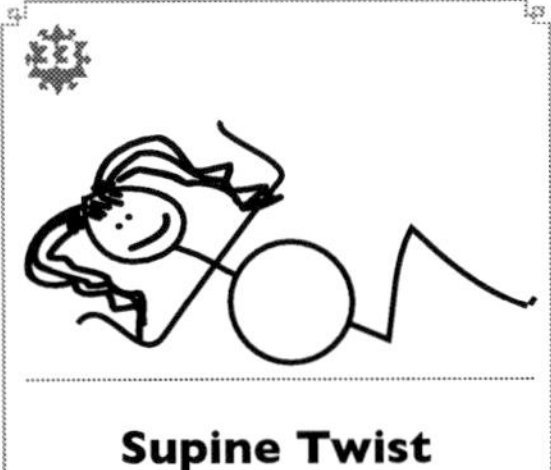

Supine Twist

Knees bent away from belly.

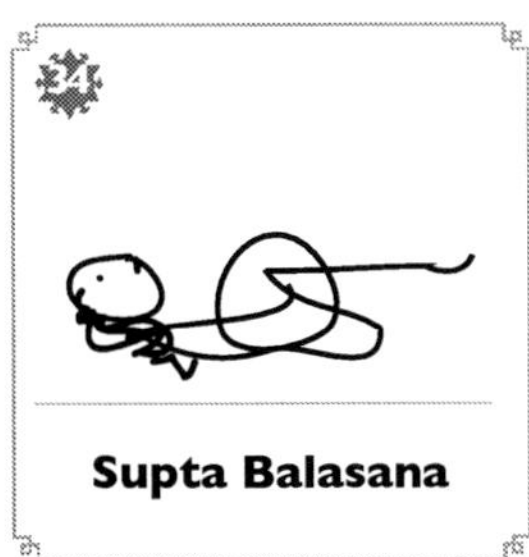

Supta Balasana

Lift head above heart after 4th month.

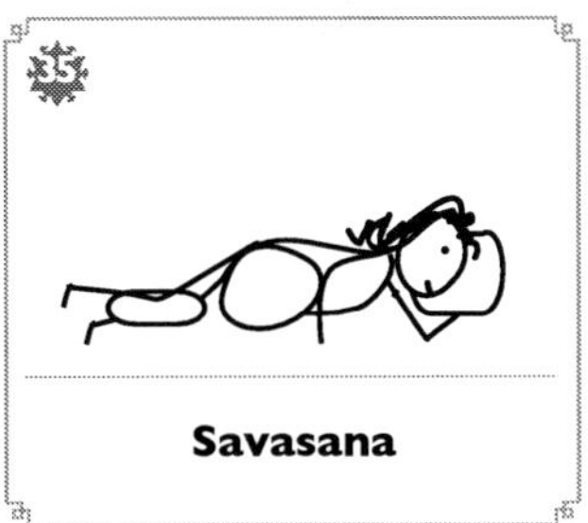

Savasana

With props on left side and between legs.

Restorative Sequence

Prenatal restorative postures encourage deep relaxation and stress relief, which support a pregnant woman in maintaining optimal health and avoiding injury and illness. If any of the poses feel uncomfortable, a pregnant woman should discontinue practicing them and try again another day. (Judith Lasater's book *Relax and Renew* is a great resource for restorative pose set ups.)

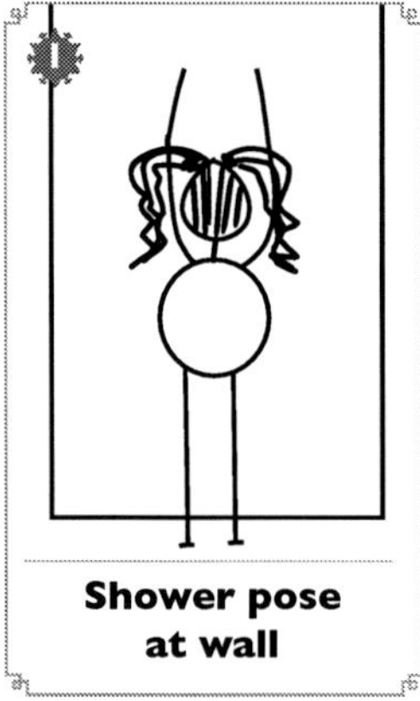

Shower pose at wall

(1-2 minutes): Facing the wall with arms stretched up, hands on wall.

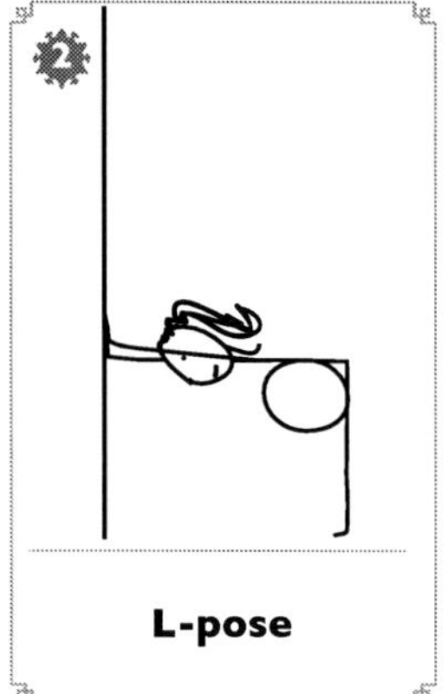

L-pose

(1-2 minutes): Relieves tension in back muscles, moves uterus up and forward out of pelvis, moves fetus away from nerves on back side of body, which may relieve spinal nerve pain.

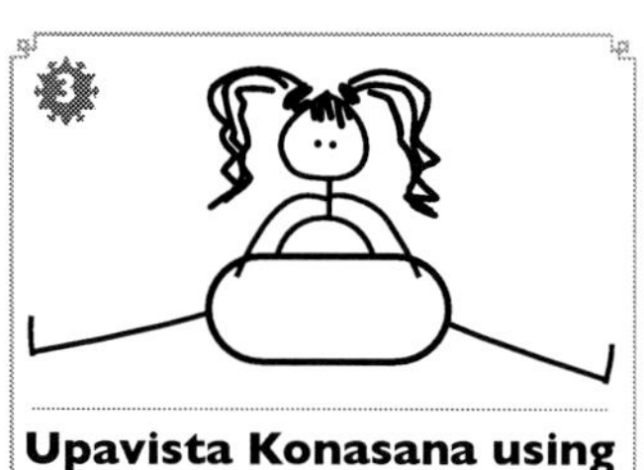

Upavista Konasana using a folding chair or several bolsters

(3-5 minutes): Soothes nervous system, releases hamstrings, quiets mind, relieves headaches and insomnia.

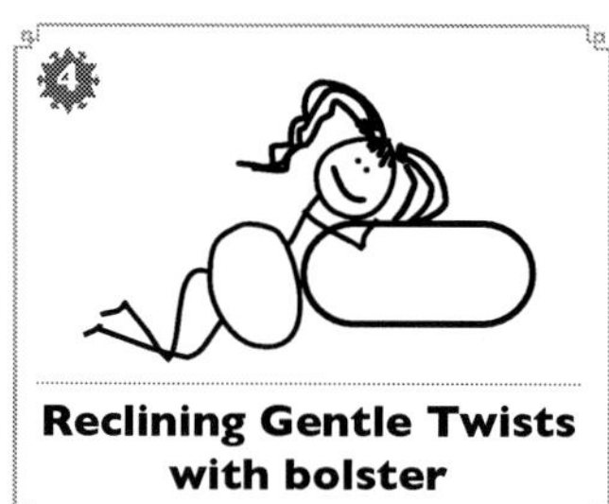

Reclining Gentle Twists with bolster

(30 seconds-2 minutes per side): Relieves stress on back muscles, stretches intercostal muscles between ribs, which may aid in breathing.

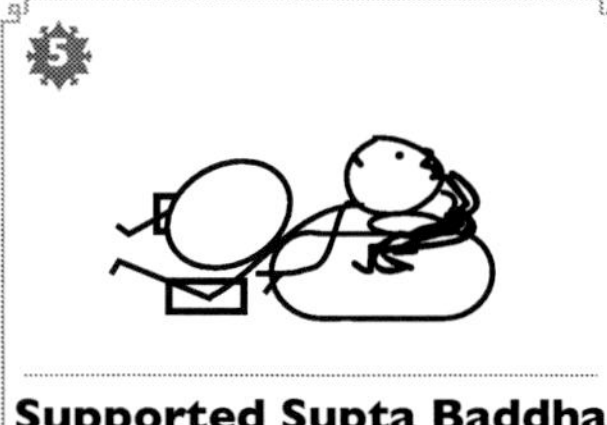

Supported Supta Baddha Konasana

(3-5 minutes): Deeper hip opener, benefits digestion and elimination, helps constipation, helps nasal congestion.

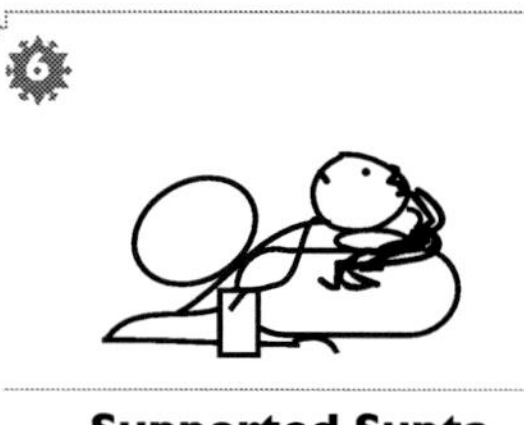

Supported Supta Virasana

(3-5 minutes): Helps relieve fatigue in legs, reduce swelling and varicose veins, relieves indigestion and nausea.

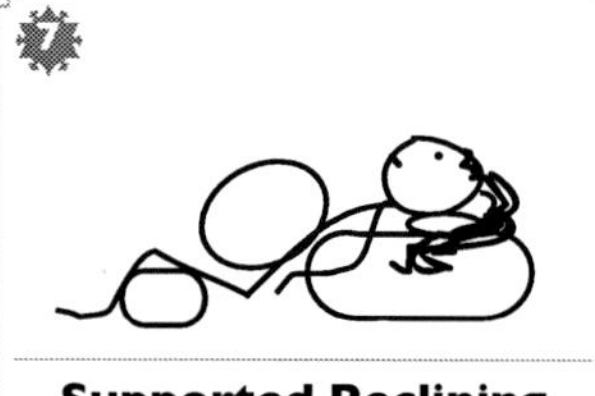

Supported Reclining Pose

(5 minutes): Calms nervous system, enhances breathing, reduces general fatigue, aids digestion and elimination.

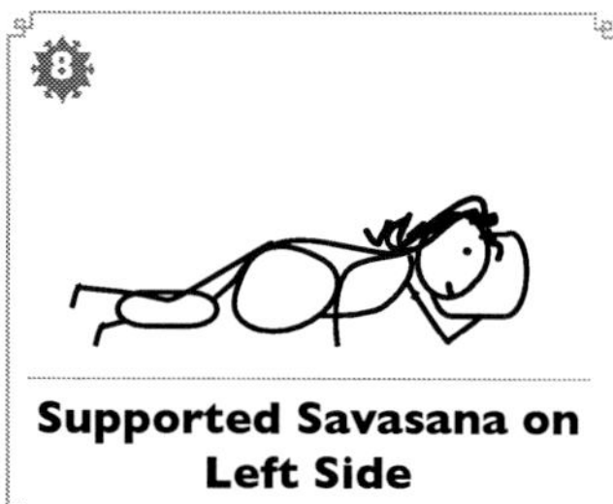

Supported Savasana on Left Side

(5-20 minutes): Relieves fatigue, nourishes baby with blood and oxygen, reduces high blood pressure.

Nausea Sequence

When it comes to nausea, take it slow and day to day. Stay longer in the poses that feel good and skip the ones that don't.

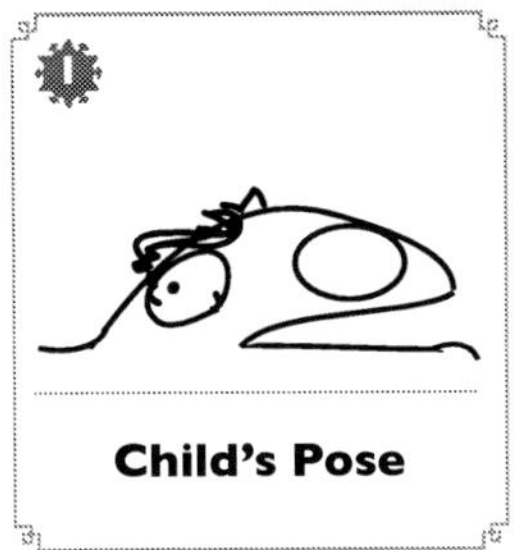

Child's Pose

5 gentle breaths.

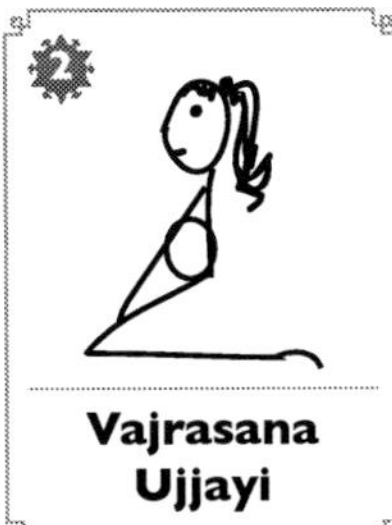

Vajrasana Ujjayi

Sit on tops of feet or blanket. Breathe 5 slow breaths.

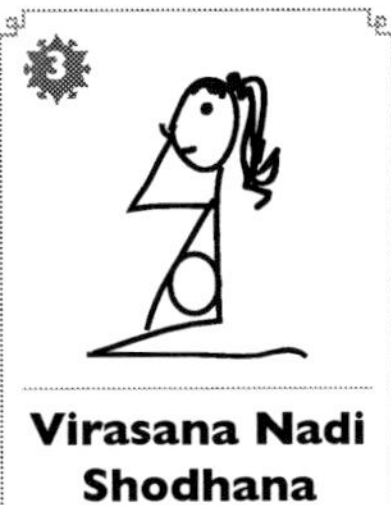

Virasana Nadi Shodhana

1 minute. Alternate nostril breathing, do not hold breath.

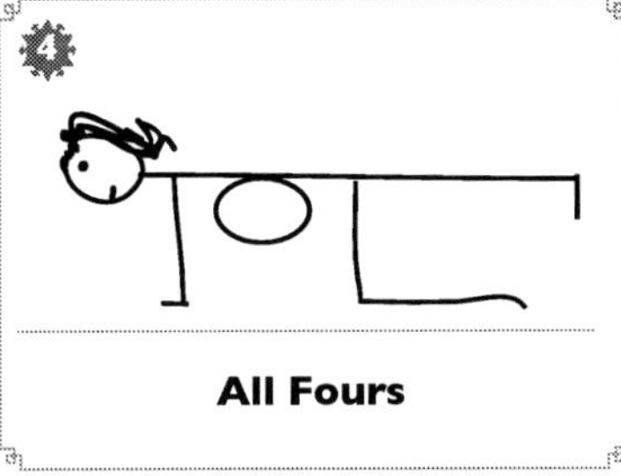

All Fours

One leg back at a time. 5 full breaths.

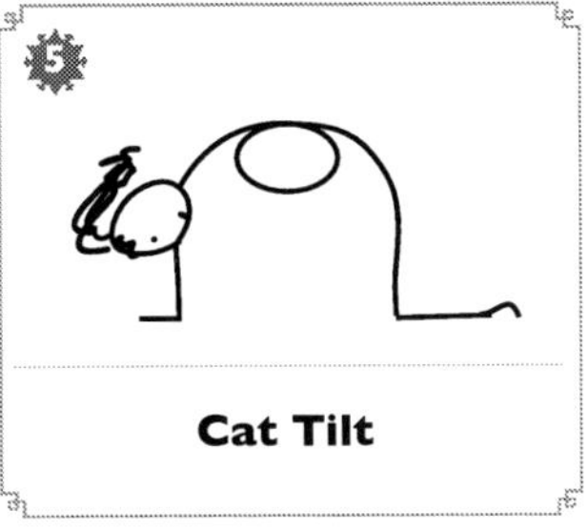

Cat Tilt

3x. Gentle movement in spine. Keep spine neutral on inhalation.

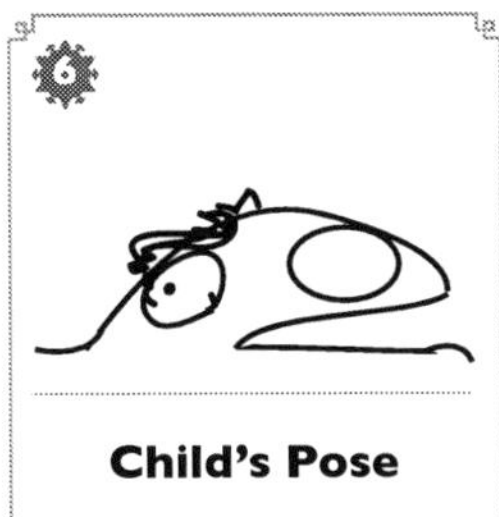

Child's Pose

5 gentle breaths.

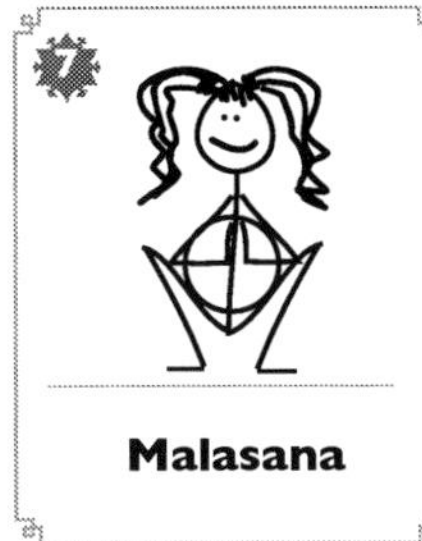

Malasana

30 seconds.

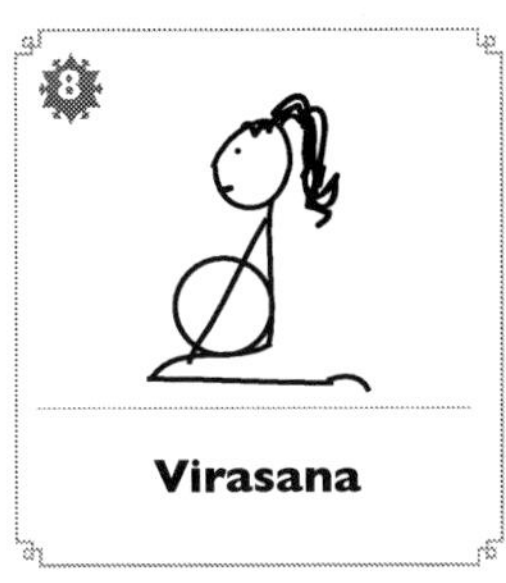

Virasana

Use block or blanket if needed. Root thighs.

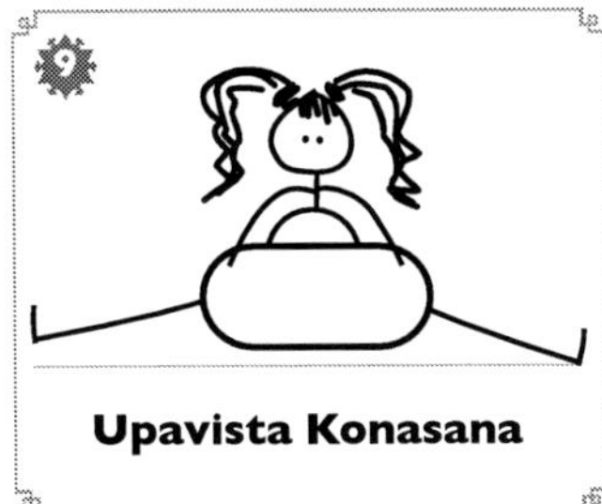

Upavista Konasana

30 seconds. Fold forward if possible, rest on bolster.

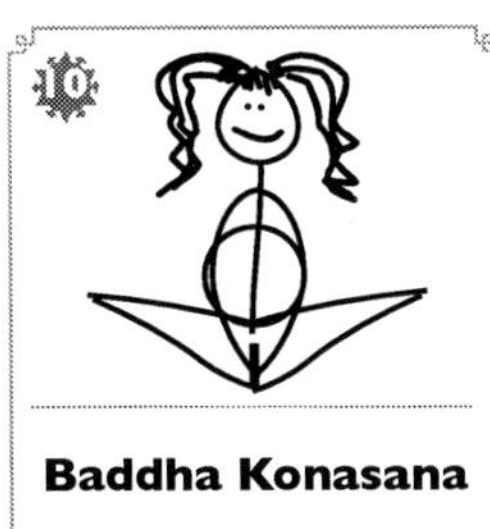

Baddha Konasana

30 seconds.

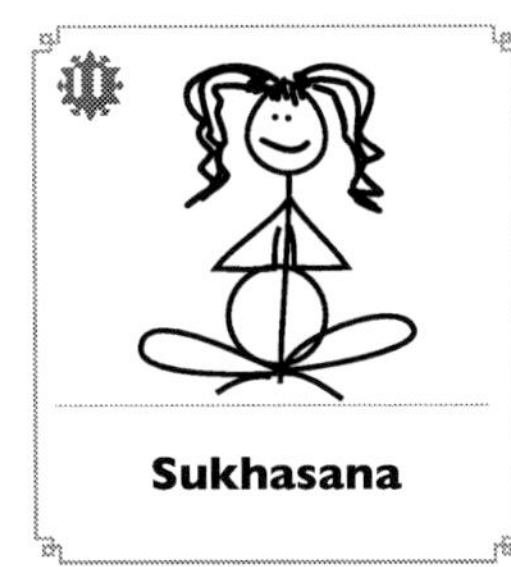

Sukhasana

5 full breaths.

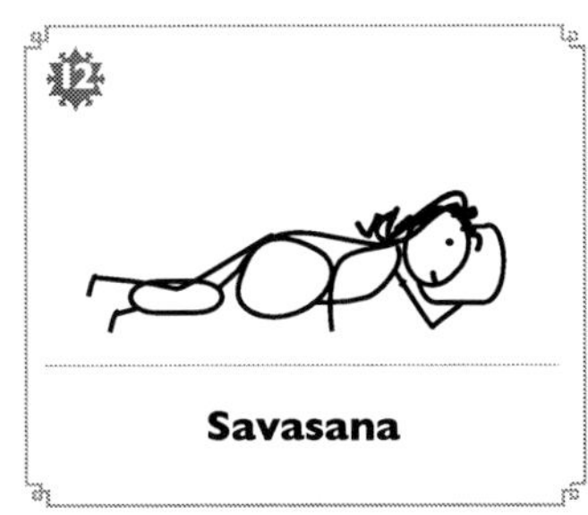

Savasana

With props on left side and between legs.

Infertility Sequence (Mixed Level)

This sequence should be done focusing on stretching the legs and rooting the femurs. New students should be with a teacher to ensure alignment.

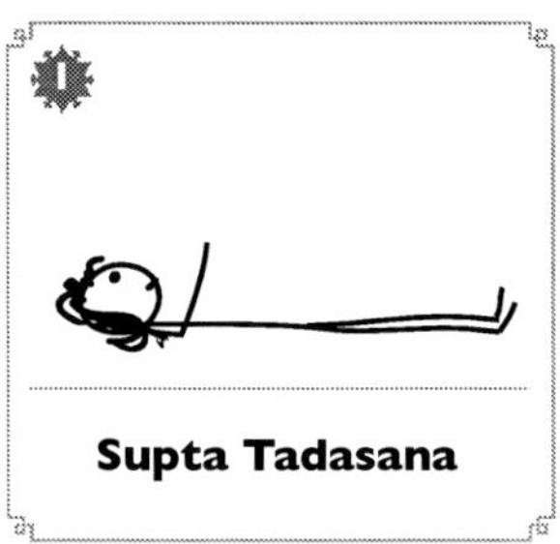

Supta Tadasana

Keep curve in lower back. Arms overhead (up and down) with breath.

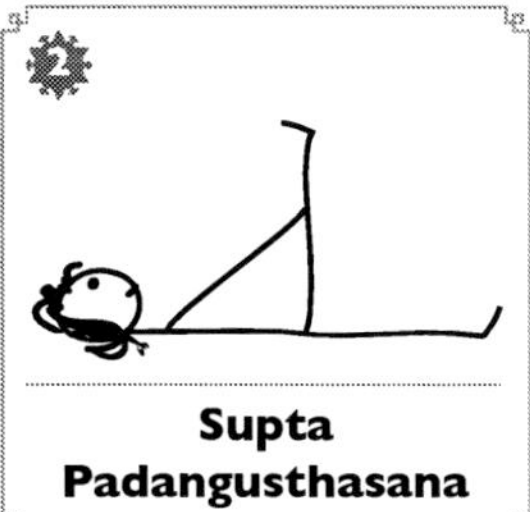

Supta Padangusthasana

Bottom leg rooted to floor, top leg straight up. Use strap if needed.

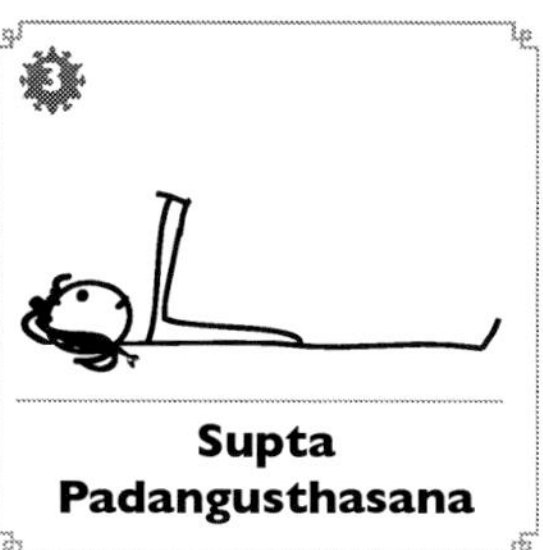

Supta Padangusthasana

Bend top knee towards floor.

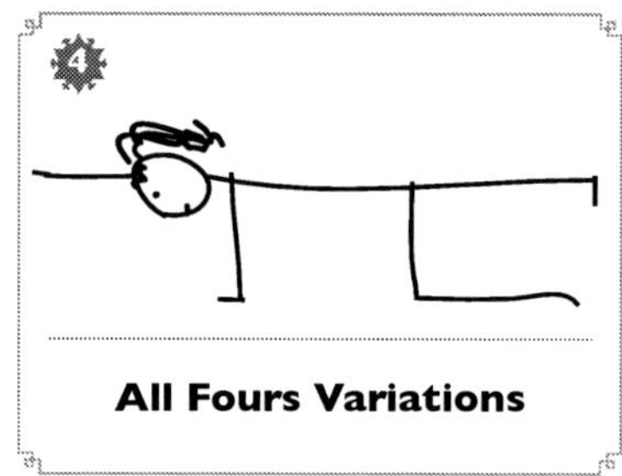

All Fours Variations

Balancing opposite arm/leg.

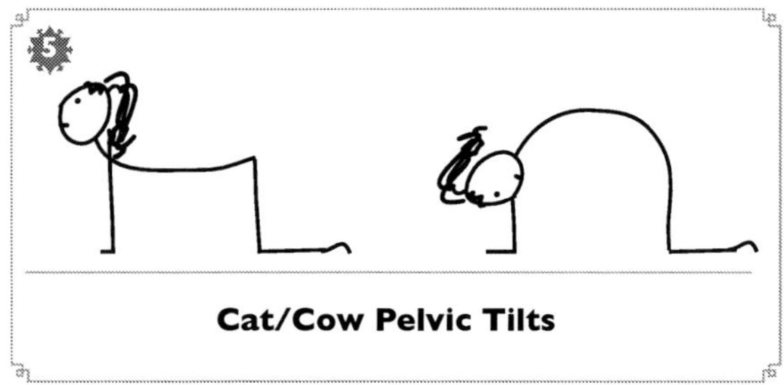

Cat/Cow Pelvic Tilts

5x. Link breath with movement.

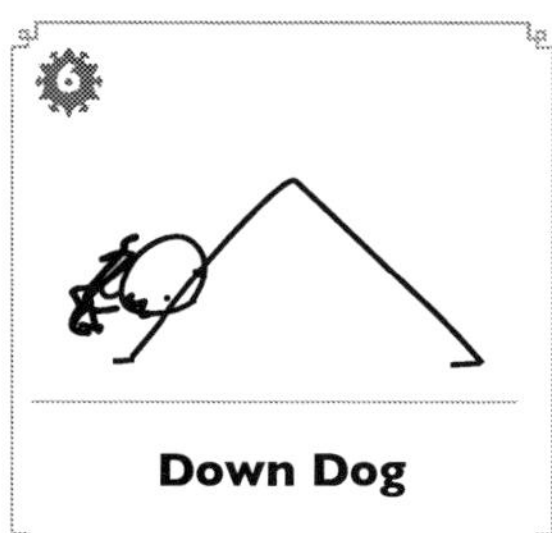

Down Dog

Uttanasana

With hands elevated on blocks if needed, root thighs back.

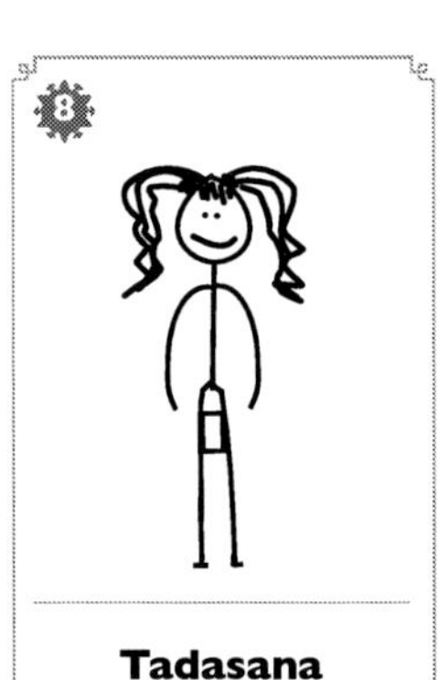

Tadasana

With block between upper inner thighs.

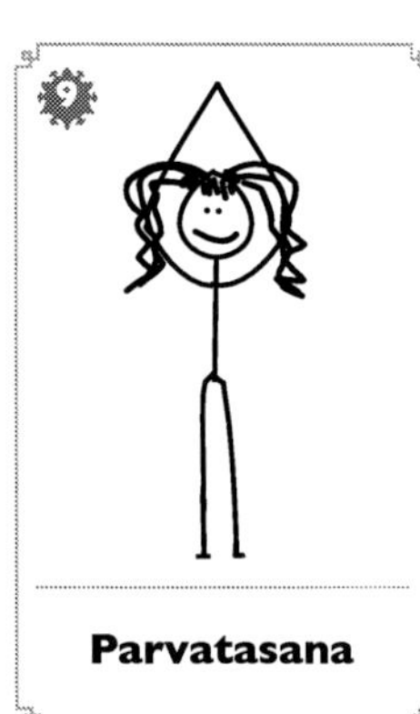

Parvatasana

Arms overhead. Root thighs back.

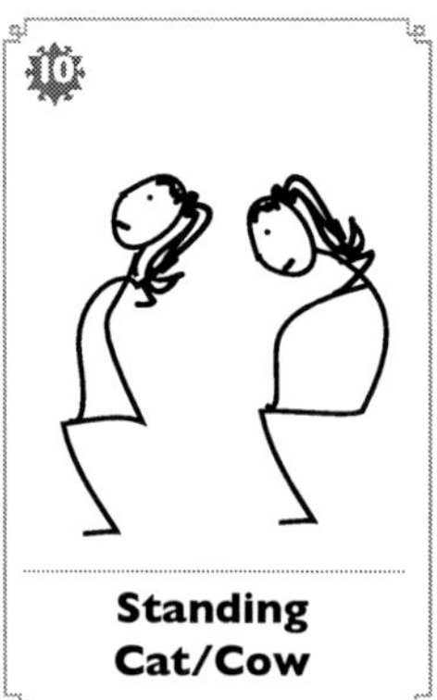

Standing Cat/Cow

Pelvic tilts.

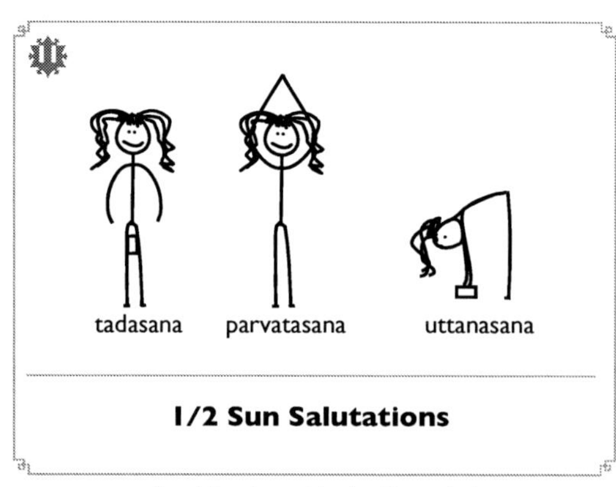

1/2 Sun Salutations

3x. Hands on blocks if needed.

...continued on next page

Infertility Sequence (Mixed Level)

...continued from page 102

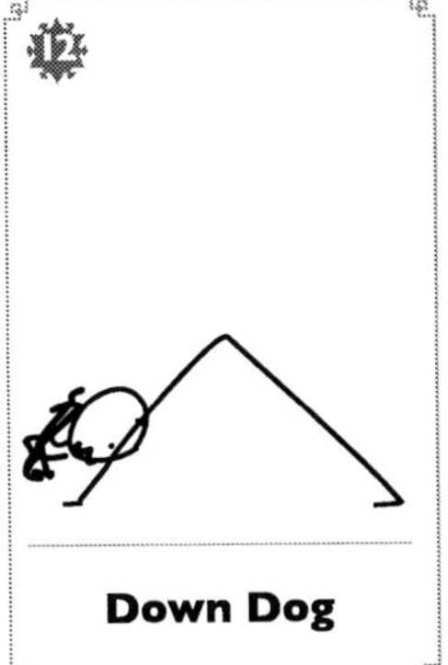

Down Dog

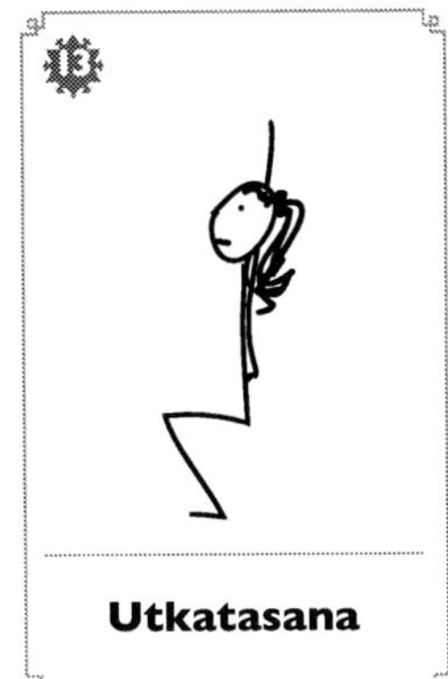

Utkatasana

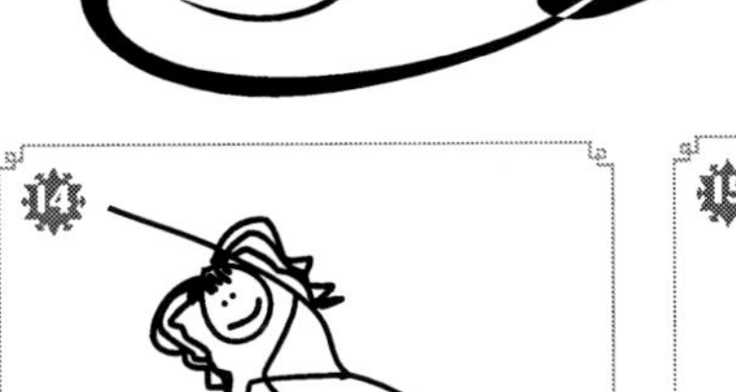

Parsvakonasana

Engage legs. Move inner thighs and sitting bones back.

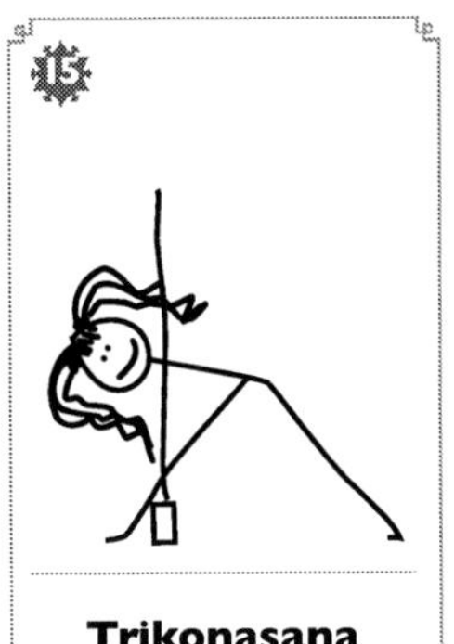

Trikonasana

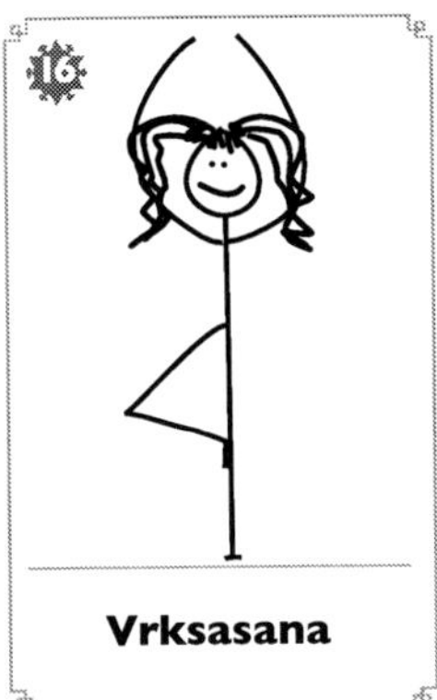

Vrksasana

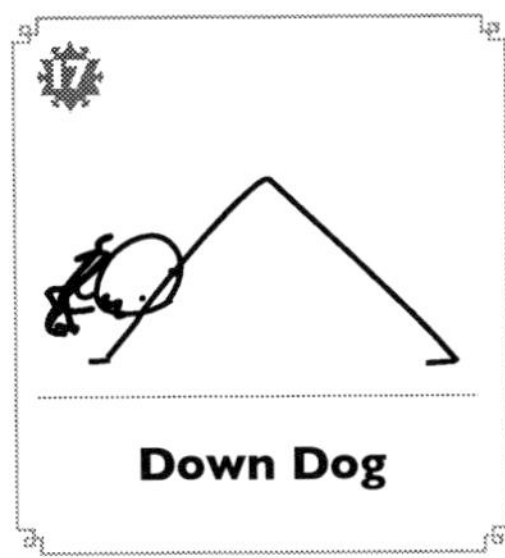

Down Dog

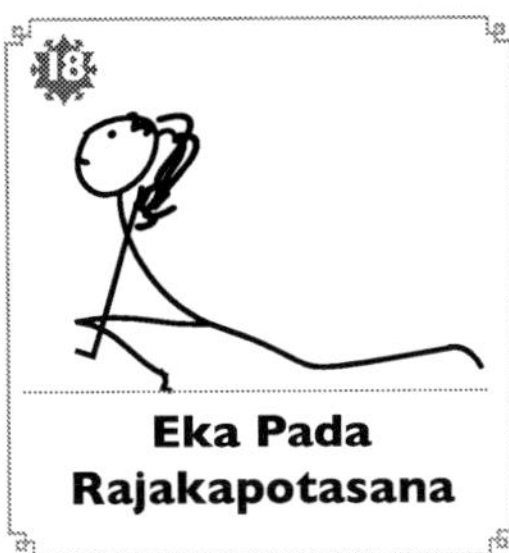

Eka Pada Rajakapotasana

Keep inner thighs engaged.

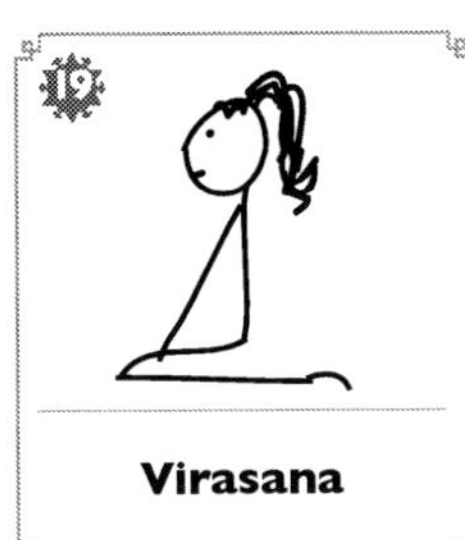

Virasana

Use block or blanket if needed.

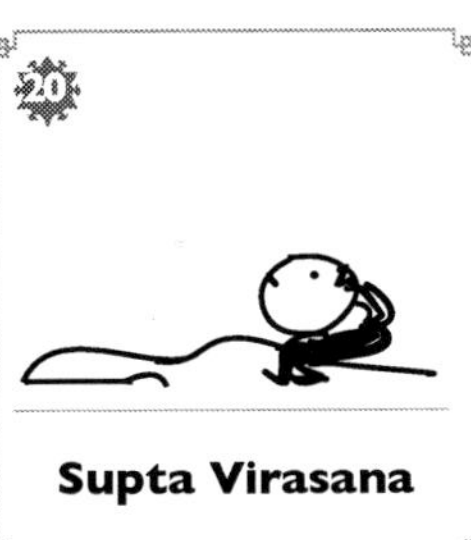

Supta Virasana

If comfortable.

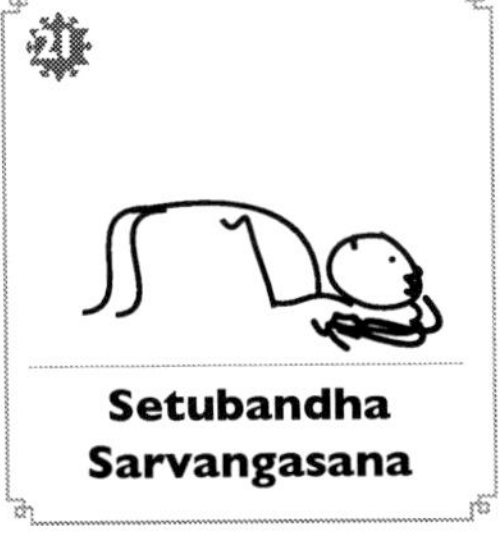
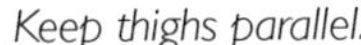

Setubandha Sarvangasana

Keep thighs parallel.

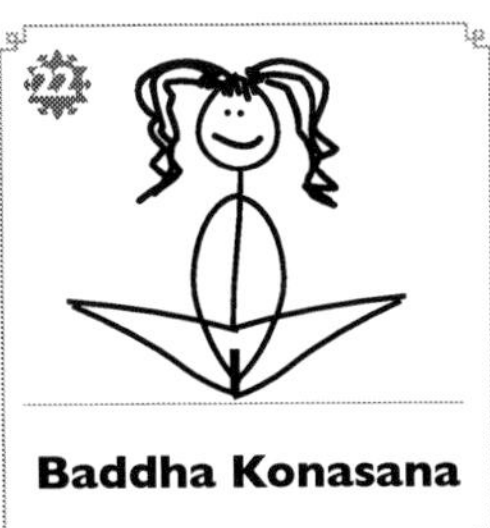

Baddha Konasana

Sit on blanket if needed.

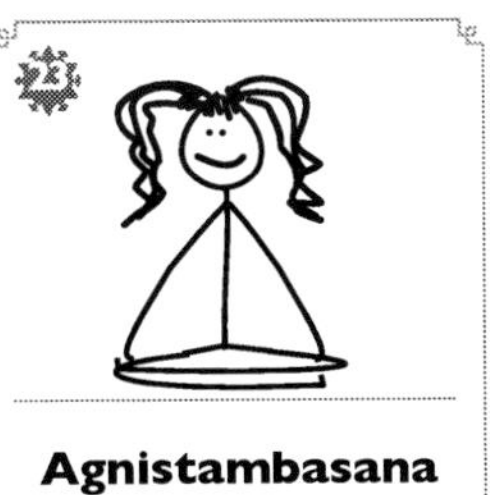

Agnistambasana

Fold forward if possible. Keep feet active.

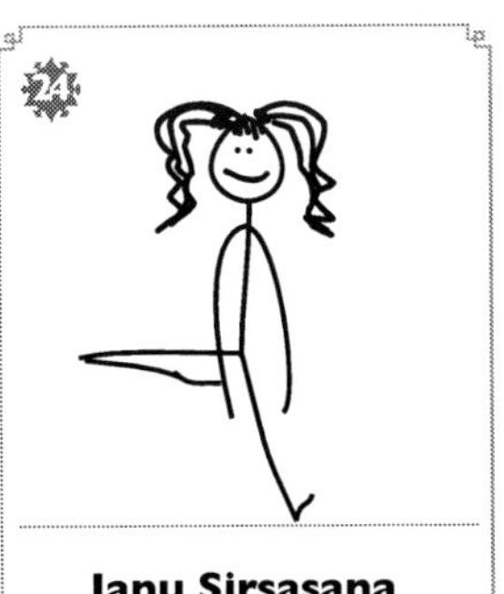

Janu Sirsasana

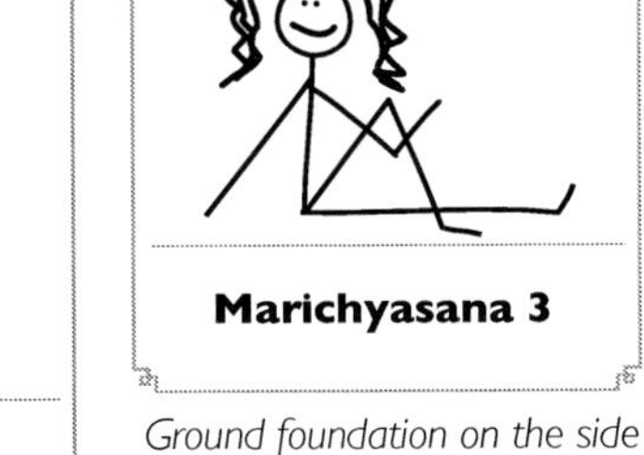

Marichyasana 3

Ground foundation on the side you are turning towards.

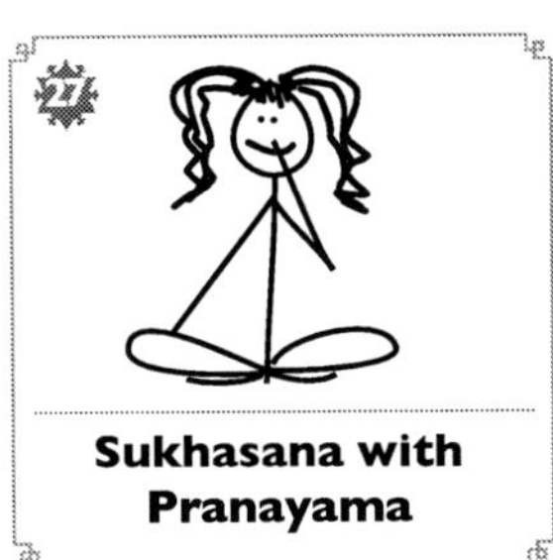

Paschimottanasana

Legs straight, root femurs.

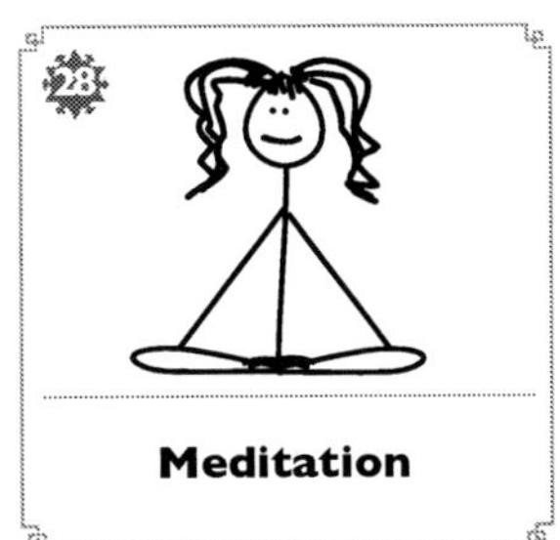

Sukhasana with Pranayama

Alternate nostril breathing.

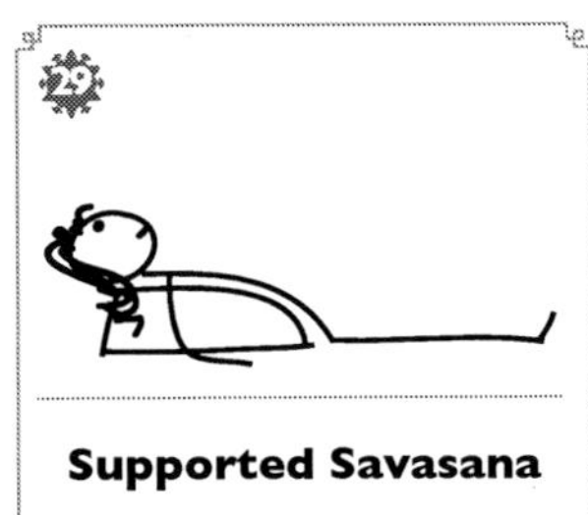

Meditation

Sit on blanket.

Supported Savasana

Allow pelvis and thighs to settle.

Postnatal Sequence

When a new mother has been advised that she can begin to exercise again, it is important to remember that this is the '4th Trimester' - she should be kind to herself as she rebuilds her strength. This practice is a wonderful transition back into movement and yoga after birth. The poses are focused on building strength, cultivating integrated actions and keeping the transverse abdominals engaged.

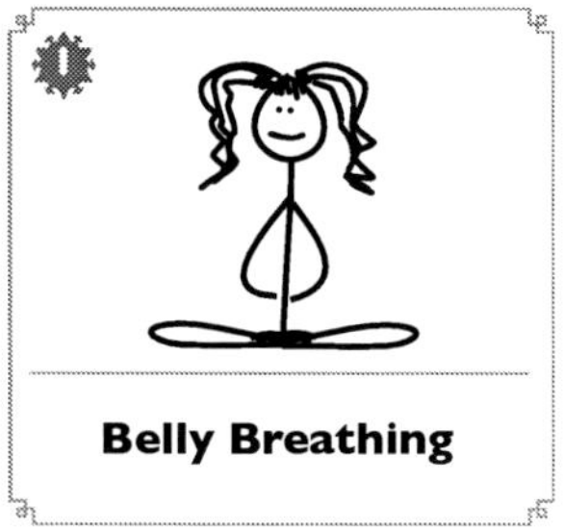

Belly Breathing

Engage the belly backwards toward the spine on exhalation. 10 deep breaths.

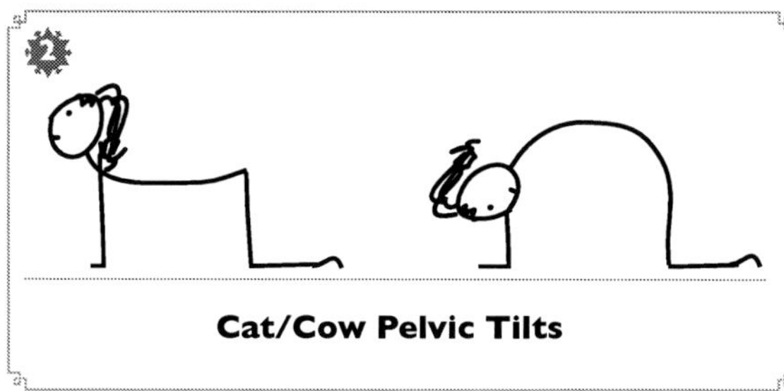

Cat/Cow Pelvic Tilts

5x. Link breath with movement.

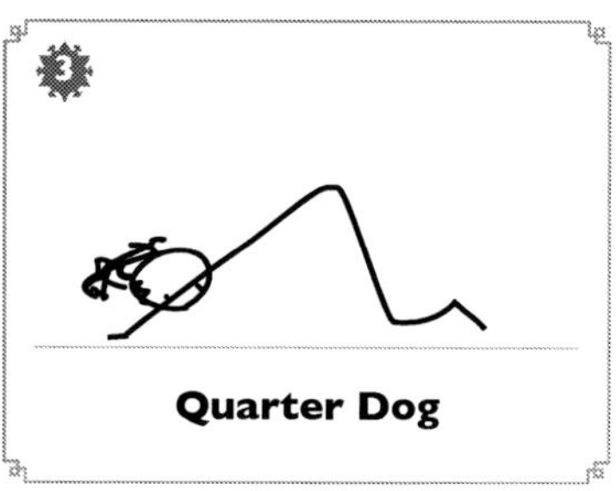

Quarter Dog

Knees on floor with down dog arms

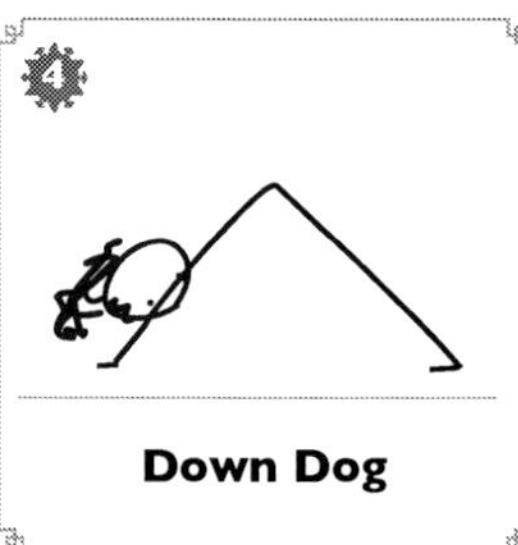

Down Dog

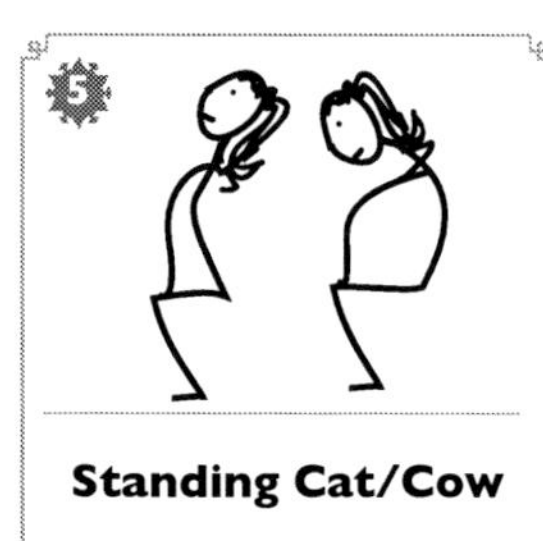

Standing Cat/Cow

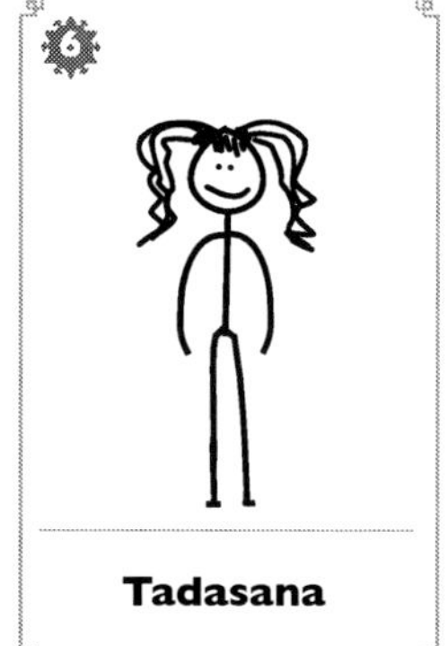

Tadasana

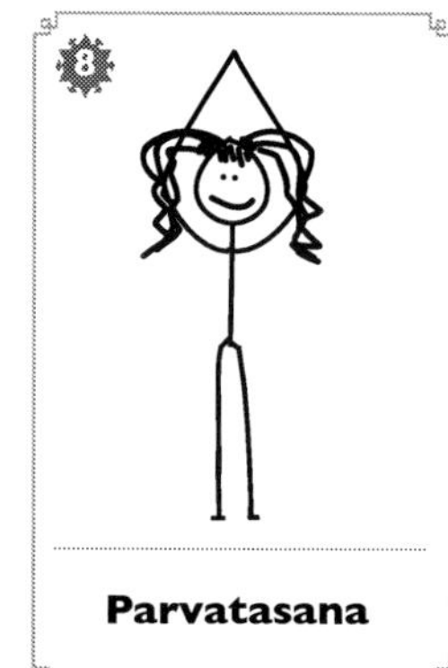

Parvatasana

Arms overhead. Root thighs back.

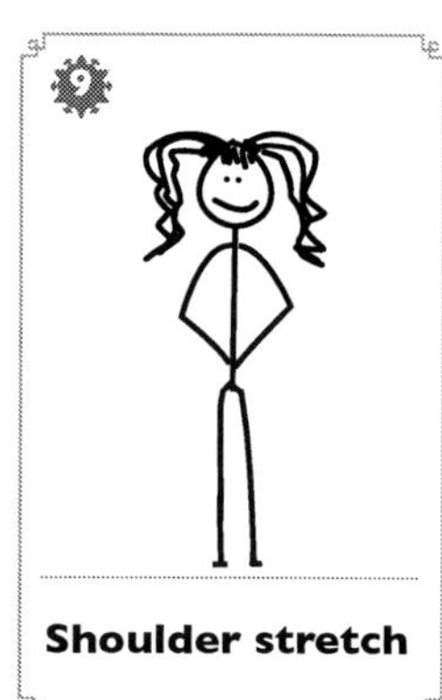

Shoulder stretch

Clasp hands behind back

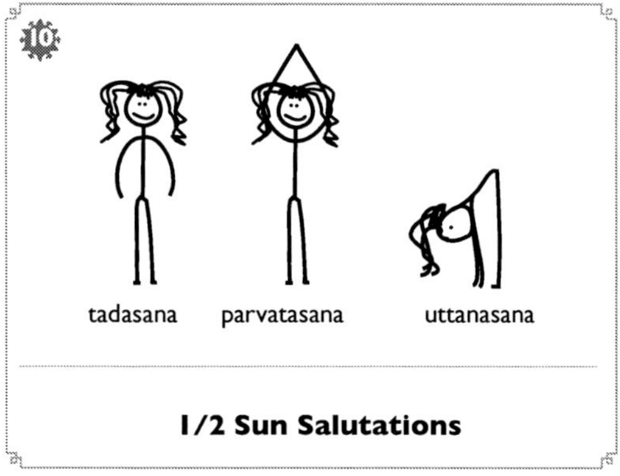

1/2 Sun Salutations

3x. Hands on blocks if needed.

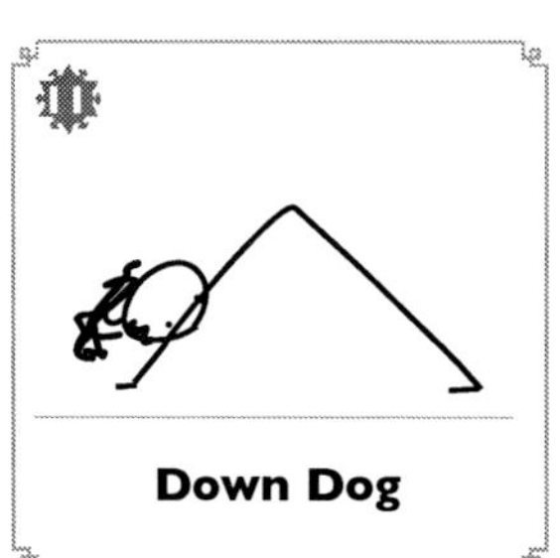

Down Dog

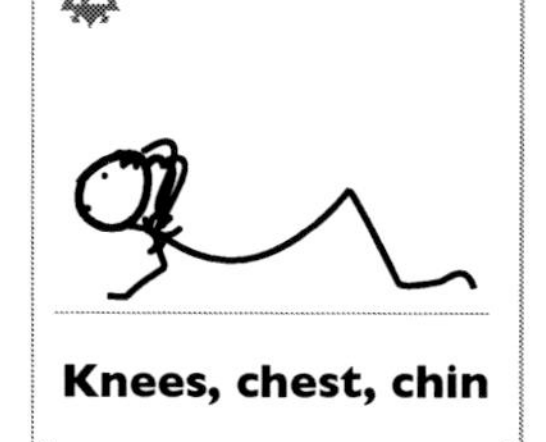

Knees, chest, chin

Shoulders and belly lift, tailbone under.

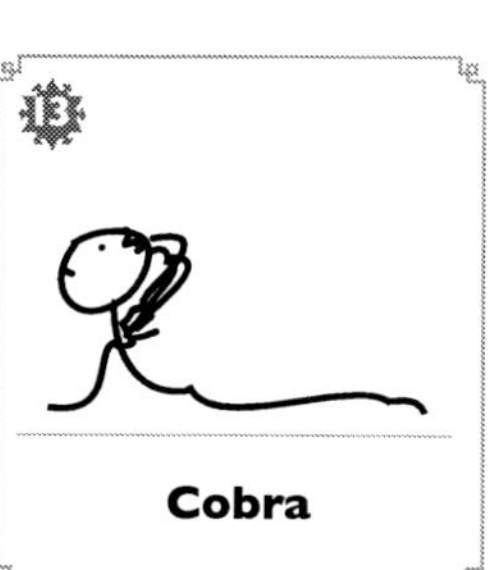

Cobra

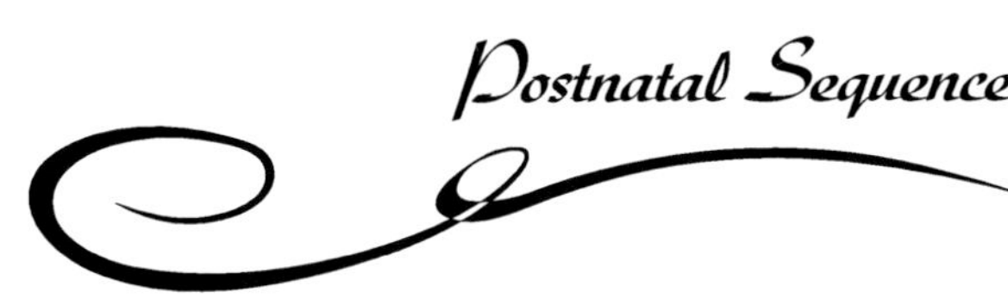

...continued from page 104

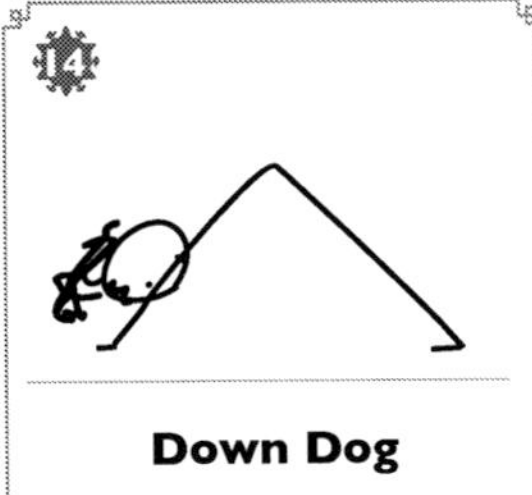

Down Dog

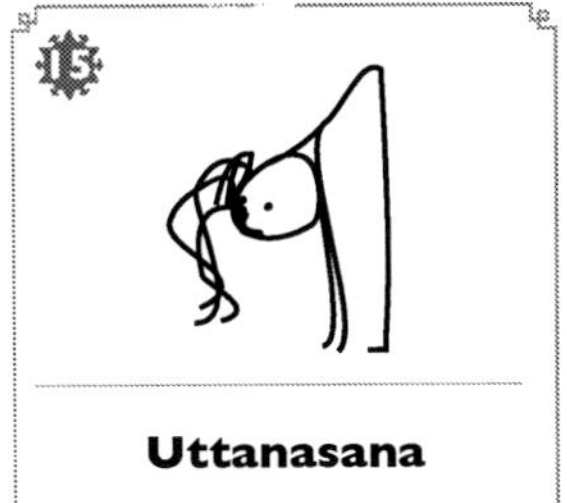

Uttanasana

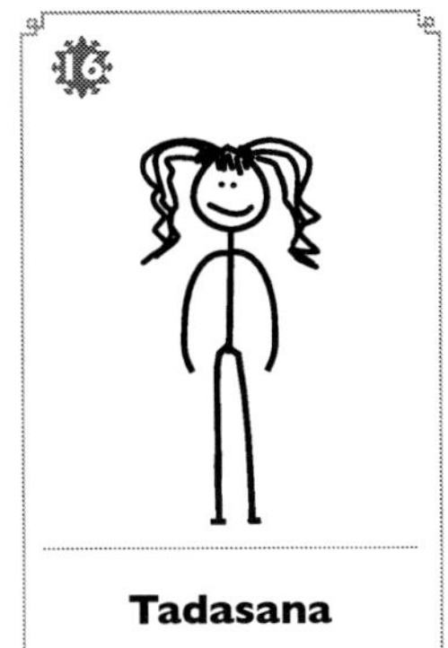

Tadasana

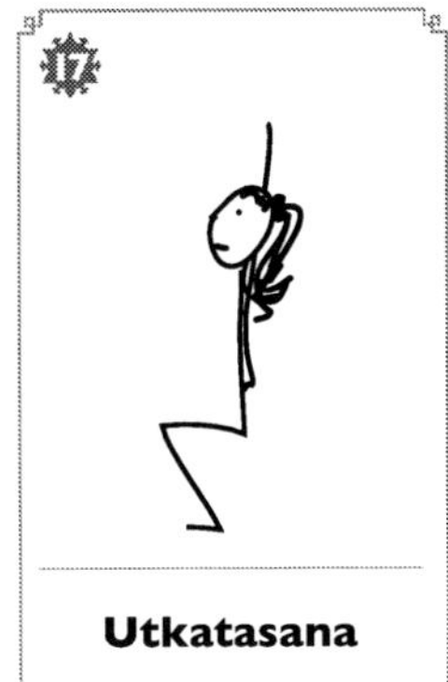

Utkatasana

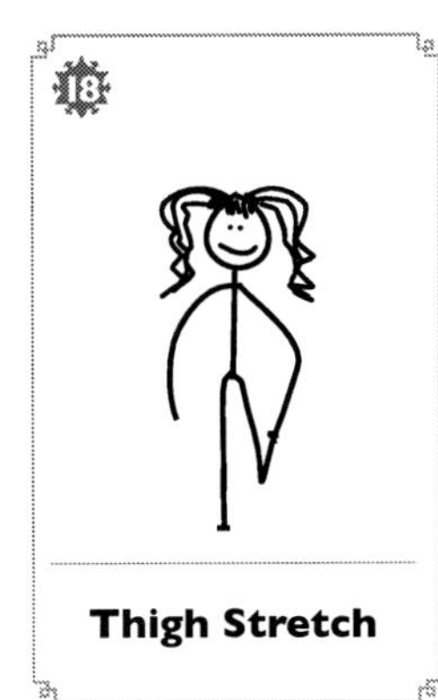

Thigh Stretch

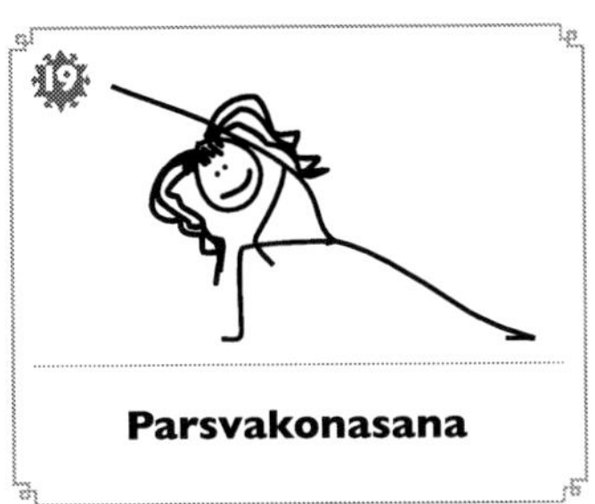

Parsvakonasana

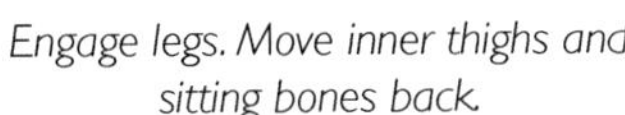

Engage legs. Move inner thighs and sitting bones back.

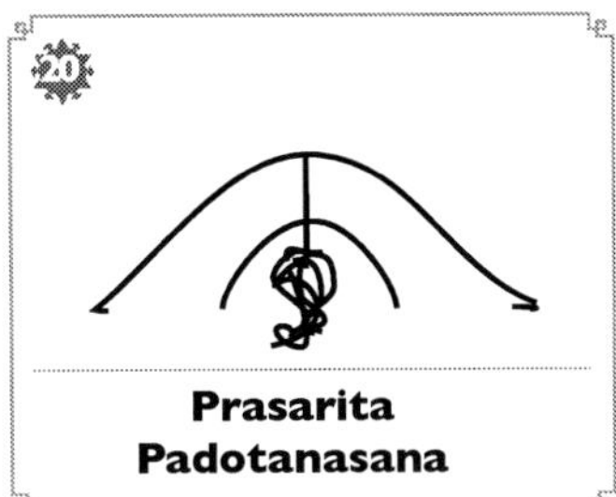

Prasarita Padotanasana

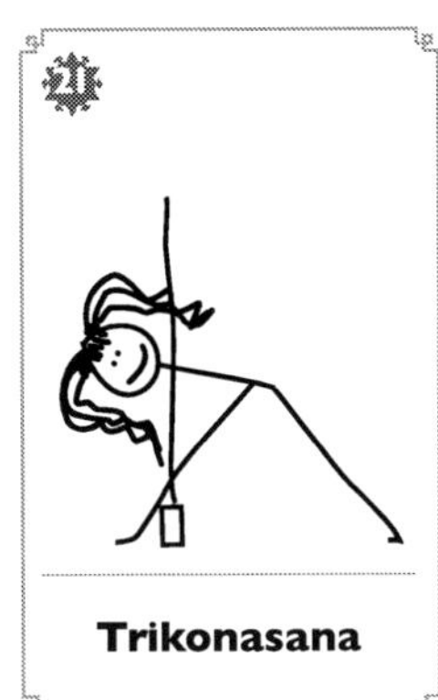

Trikonasana

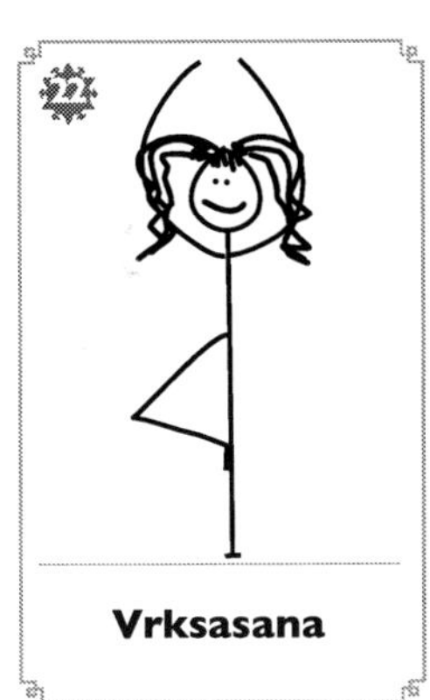

Vrksasana

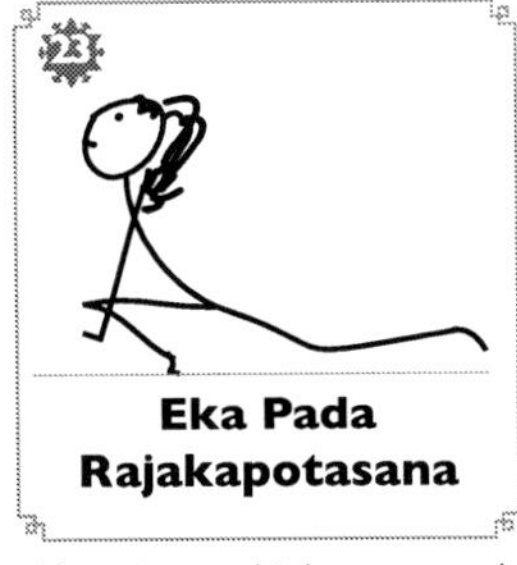

Eka Pada Rajakapotasana

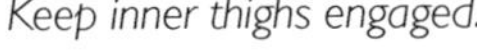

Keep inner thighs engaged.

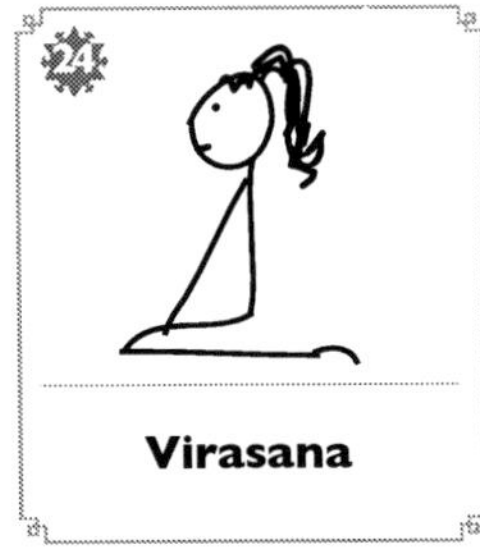

Virasana

Use block or blanket if needed.

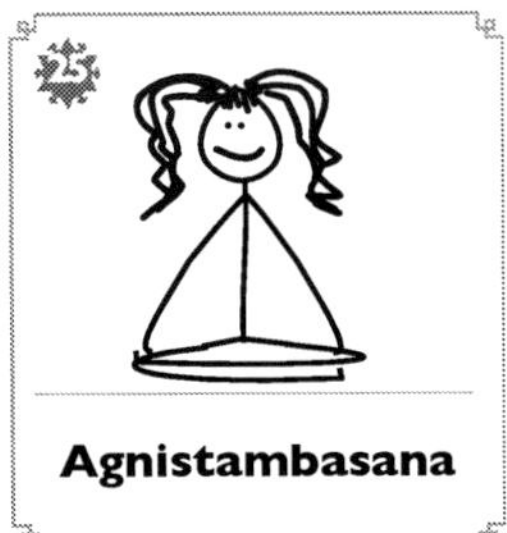

Agnistambasana

Keep feet active.

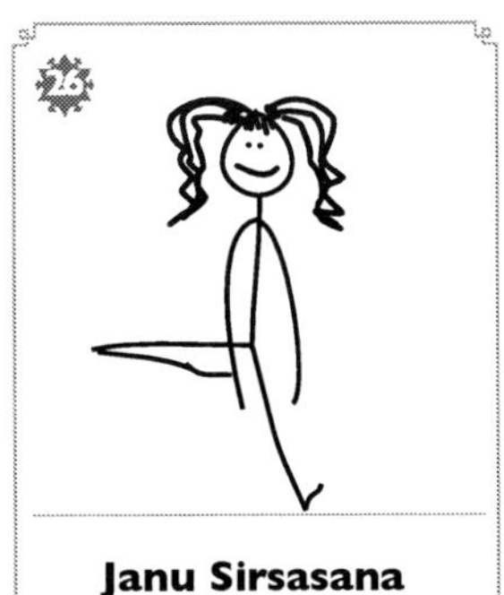

Janu Sirsasana

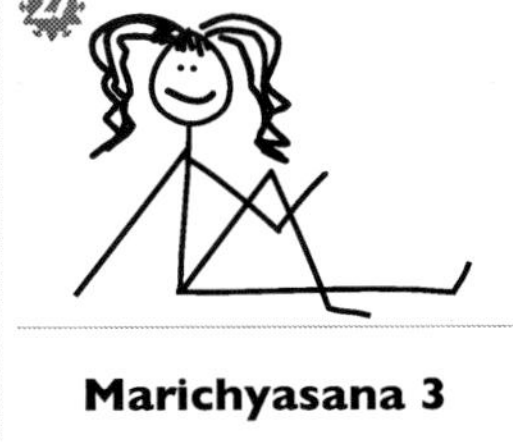

Marichyasana 3

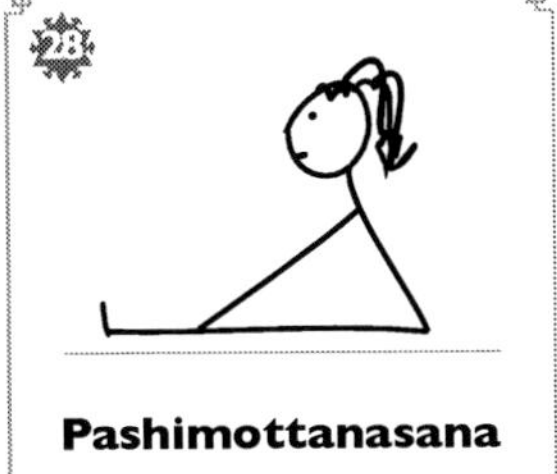

Pashimottanasana

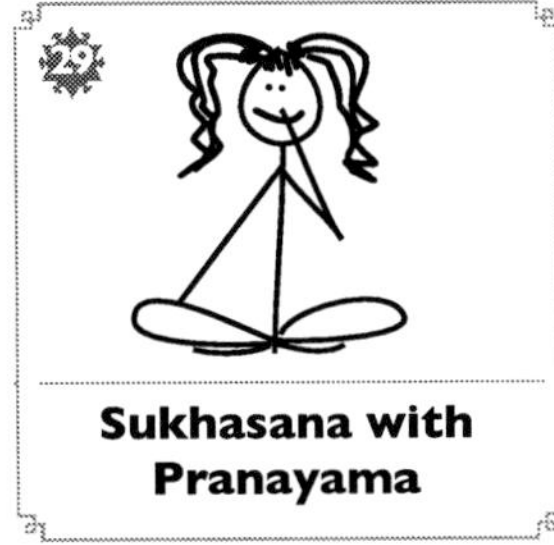

Sukhasana with Pranayama

Alternate nostril breathing.

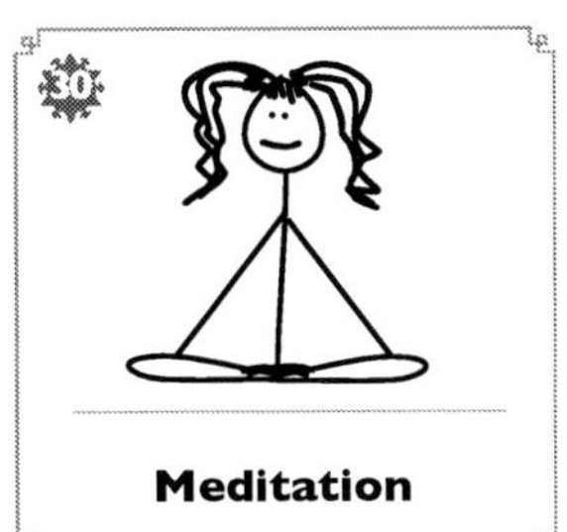

Meditation

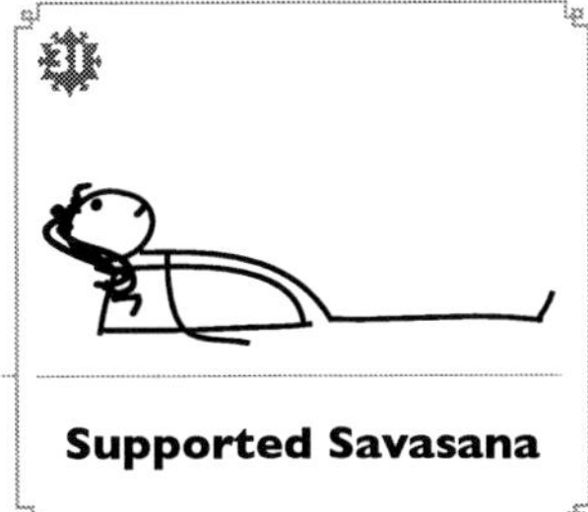

Supported Savasana

Allow pelvis and thighs to settle.

PRENATAL YOGA SYLLABUS OF ASANAS

The following is a list of yoga postures that can be practiced safely during pregnancy with the help of a qualified teacher to ensure proper alignment. All poses should be modified according to the level of practitioner and the trimester. Please make sure props are on hand, in particular blocks, blankets, and straps. Students new to yoga should avoid deep backbends, inversions, and any pose that does not feel appropriate. Advanced practitioners may want to add to this syllabus, keeping in mind the earlier section on what to be cautious of and what to avoid (see page 27).

STANDING POSES

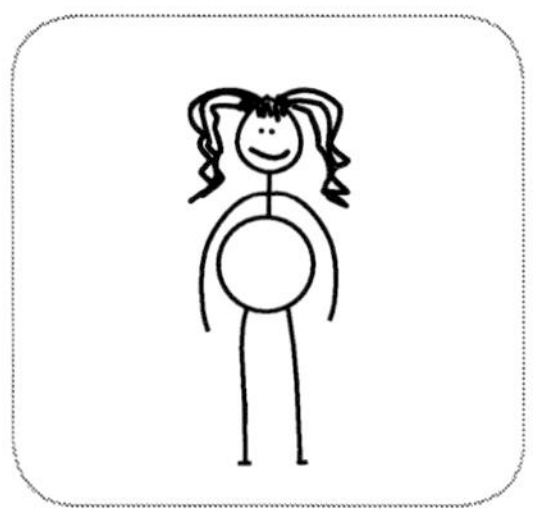

Tadasana
(mountain pose)

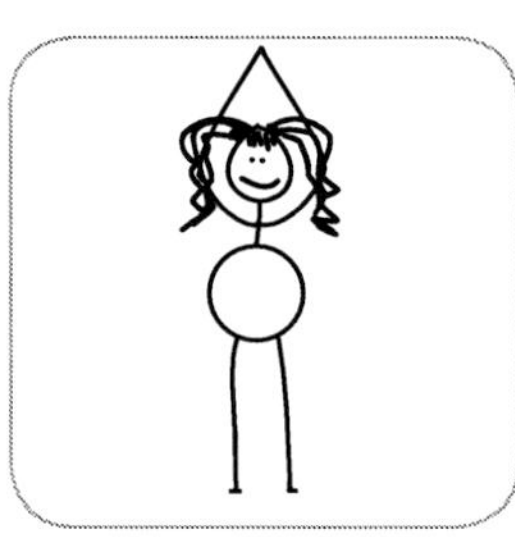

Parvatasana
(mountain pose with arms overhead)

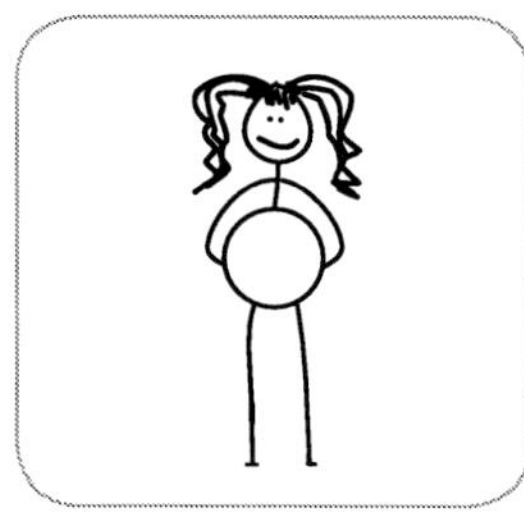

Tadasana Variation
(mountain pose with hands clasped behind back)

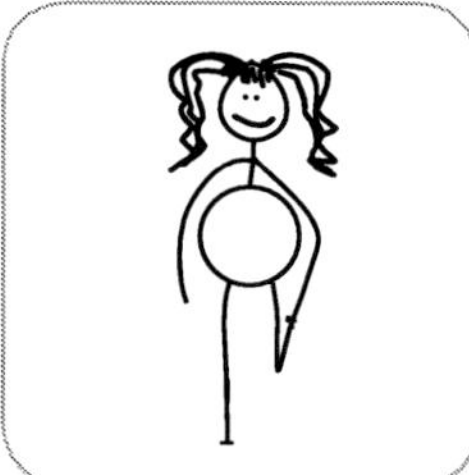

Standing Thigh Stretch

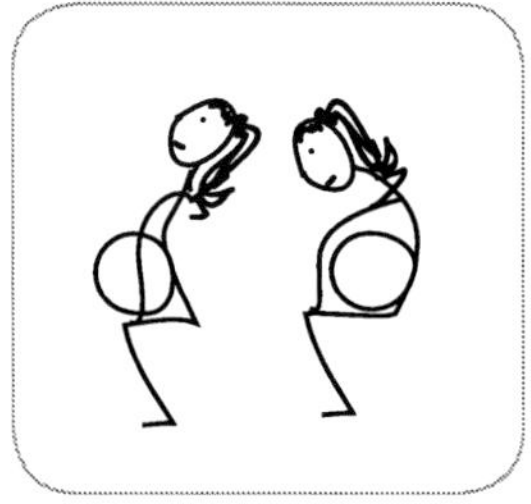

Standing Cat/Cow

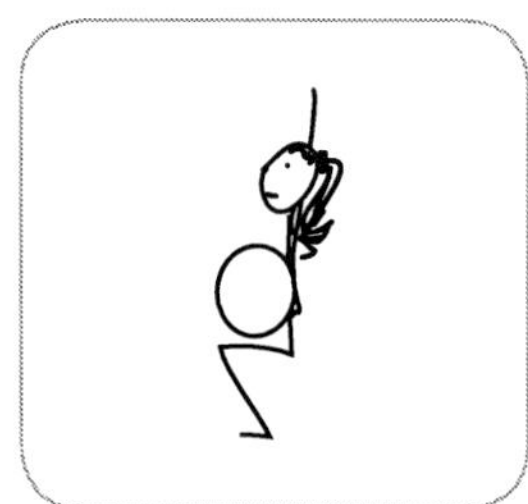

Utkatasana
(chair pose)

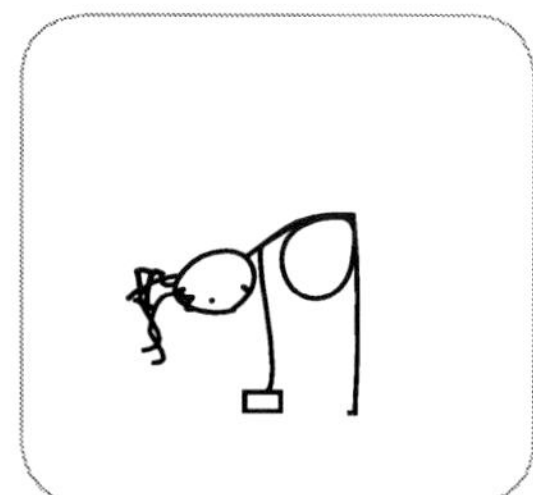

Uttanasana
(standing forward bend pose)

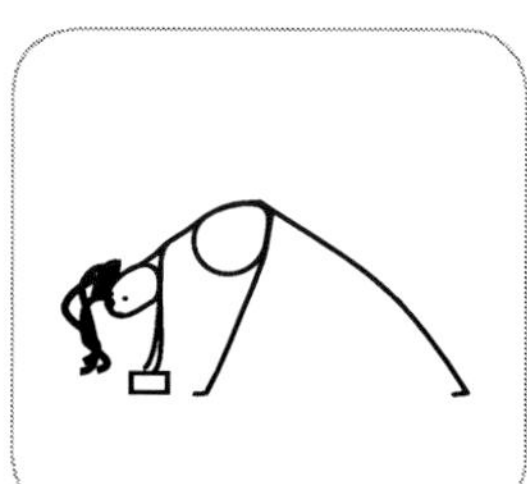

Parsvottanasana
(pyramid pose)

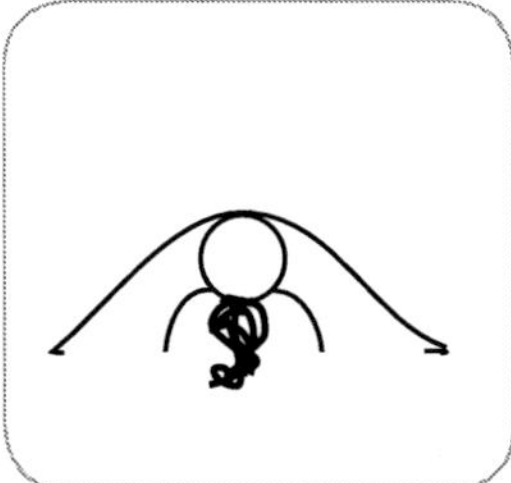

Prasarita Padottanasana
(wide-legged standing forward bend)

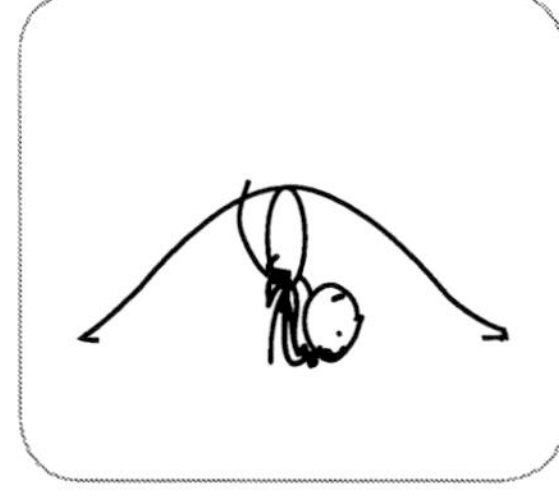

Parivrtta Prasarita Padottanasana
(twisting wide-legged standing forward bend)

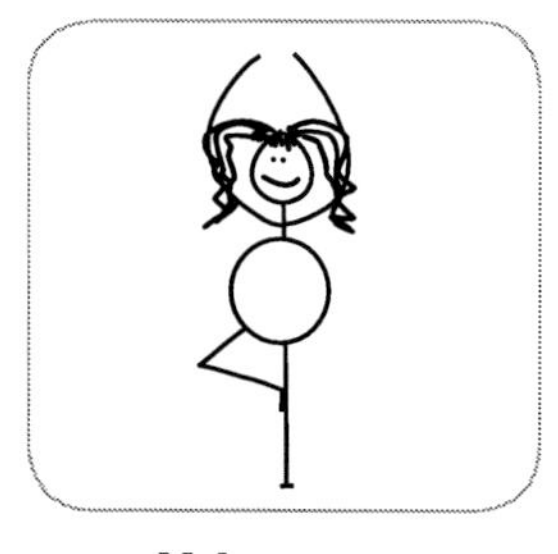

Vrksasana
(tree pose)

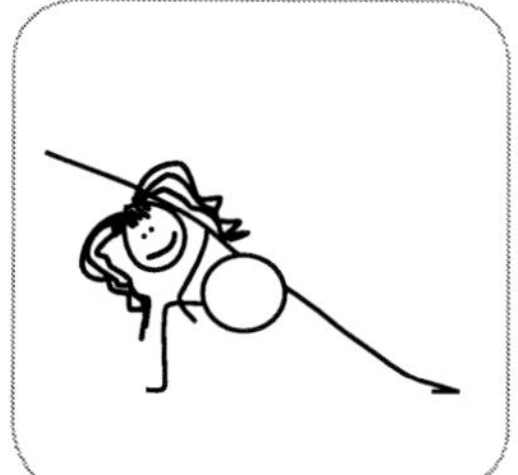

Parsvakonasana
(extended side angle pose)

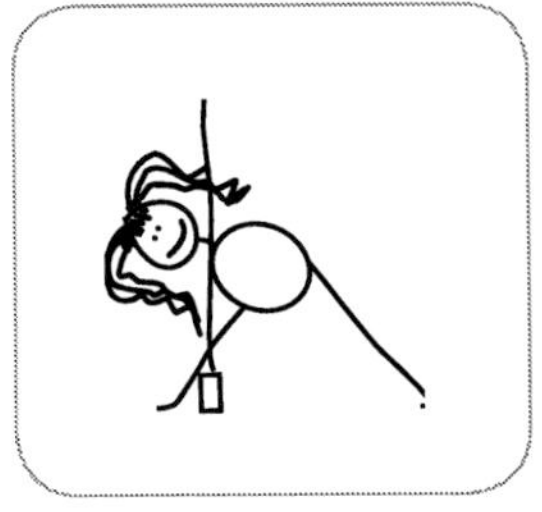

Trikonasana
(triangle pose)

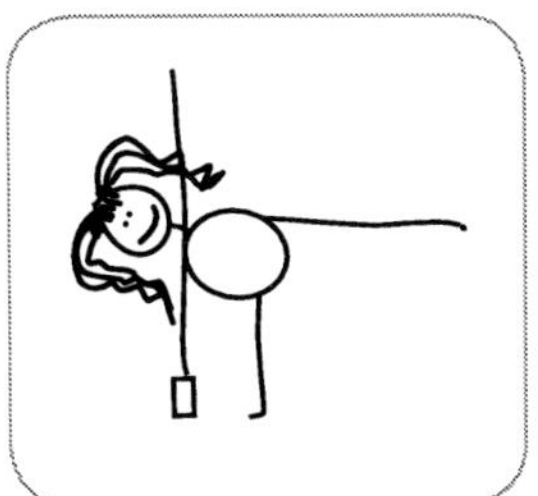

Ardha Chandrasana
(half moon pose)

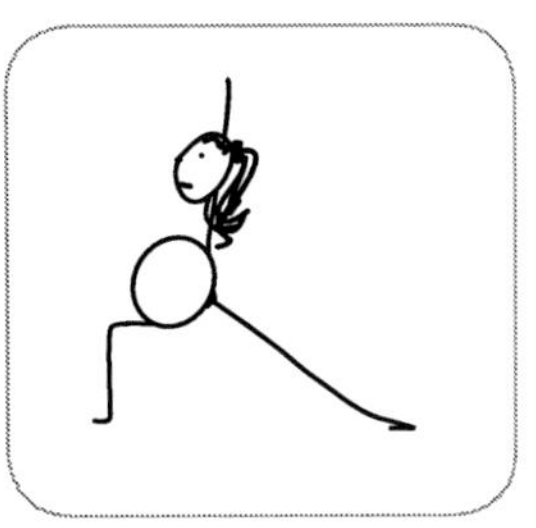

Virabhadrasana 1
(warrior one pose)

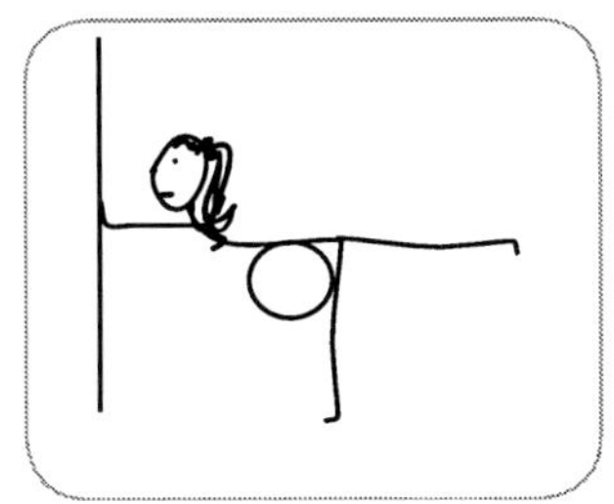

Virabhadrasana 3
(warrior three pose)

SITTING POSES, FORWARD BENDS, AND HIP OPENERS

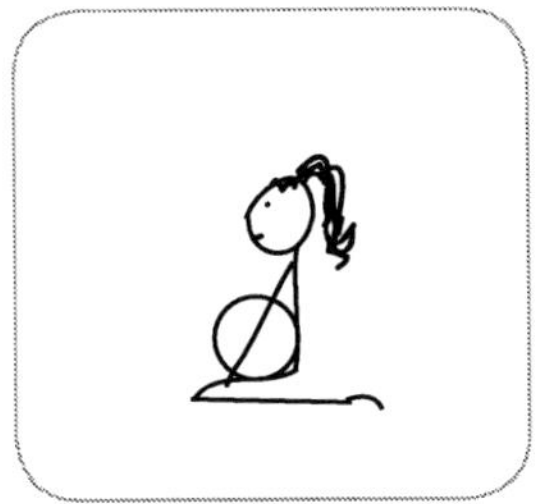

Virasana
(hero pose)

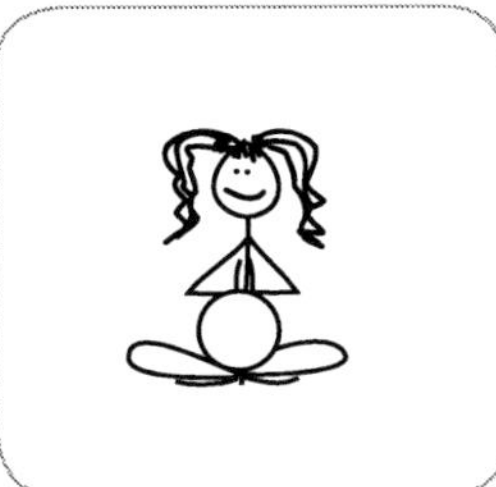

Sukhasana
(easy pose)

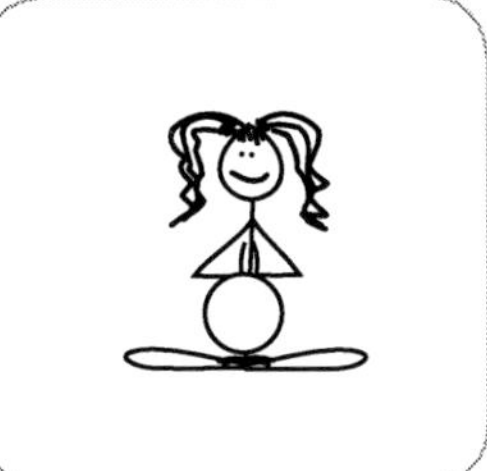

Siddhasana
(accomplished pose)

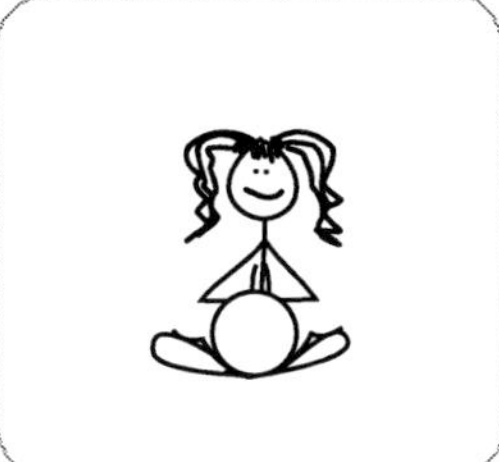

Padmasana
(lotus pose)

Baddha Konasana
(cobbler's pose)

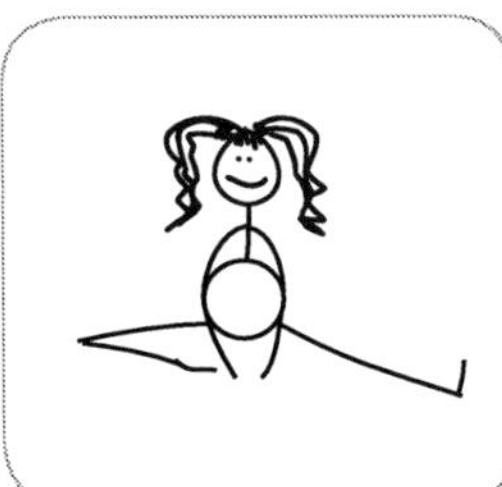

Janu Sirsasana
(modified
head to knee pose)

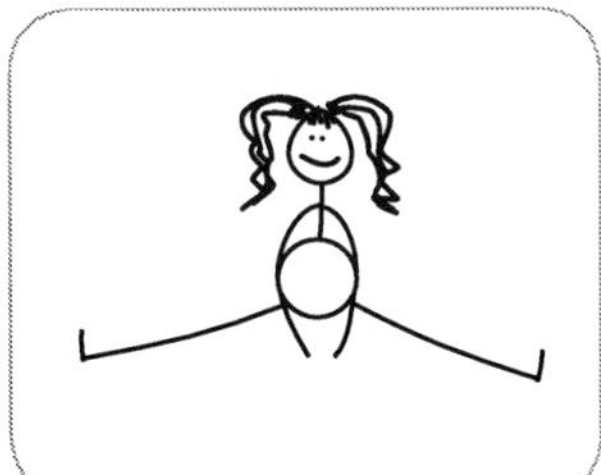

Upavista Konasana
(seated wide-angle
forward bend pose)

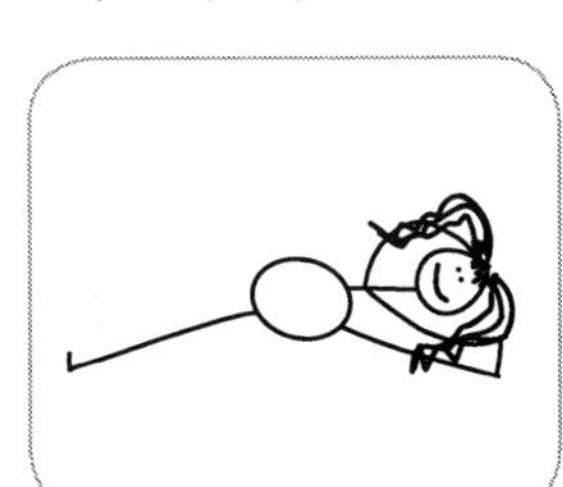

**Parivrtta Upavista
Konasana**
(revolved seated wide-angle
forward bend pose)

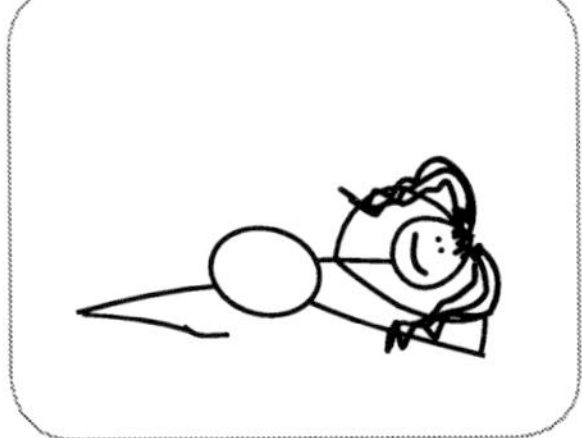

**Parivrtta Janu
Sirsasana**
(modified revolved head
to knee pose)

Agnistambasana
(firelog pose)

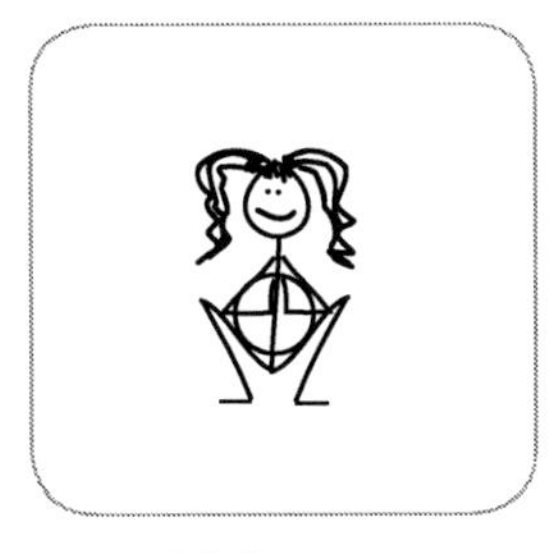

Malasana
(garland pose)

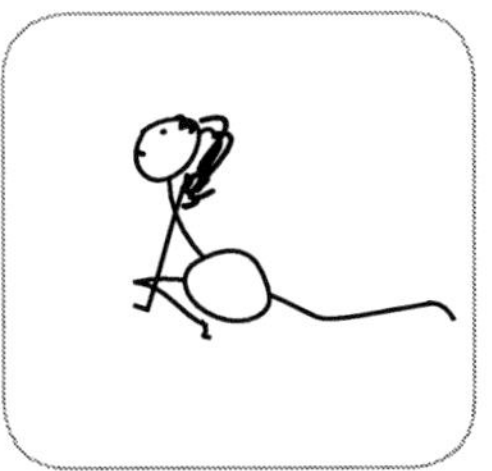

**Eka Pada
Rajakapotasana Prep**
(pigeon prep pose)

INVERSIONS AND HAND BALANCINGS

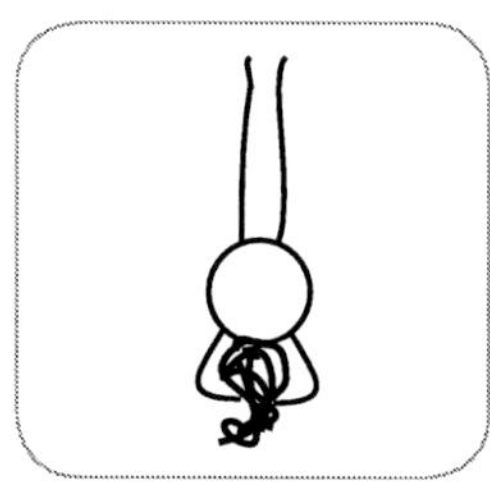

Sirsasana
(headstand pose)

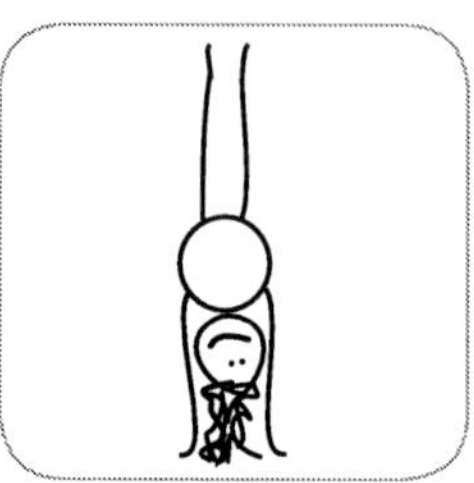

Adho Mukha Vrksasana
(handstand pose)

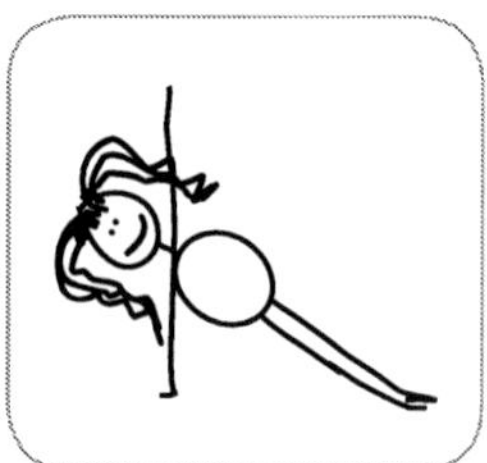

Vasisthasana
(side plank pose)

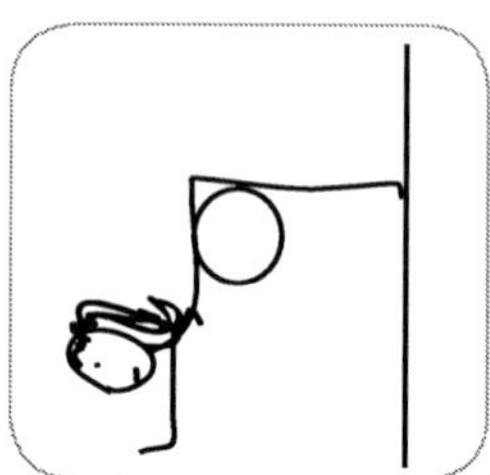

Inverted L-Pose

BACKBENDS

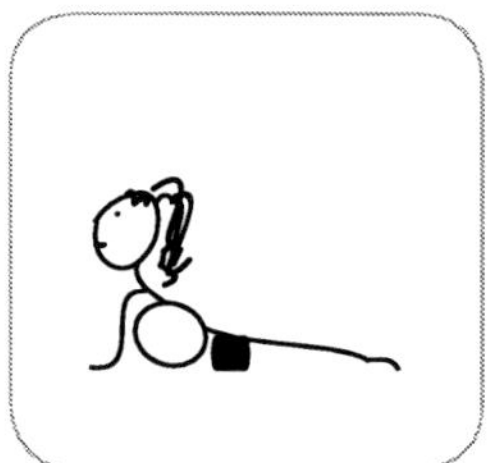

Bhujangasana
(cobra pose
with bolster)

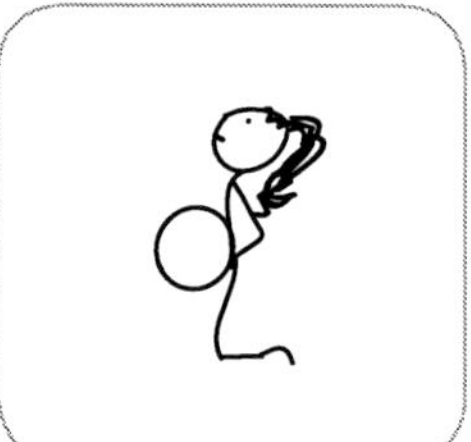

Ustrasana
(camel pose)

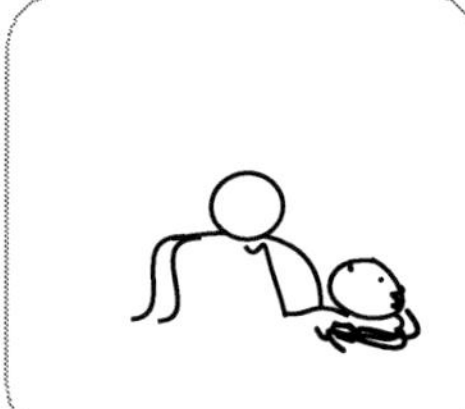

Setubandha Sarvangasana
(bridge pose)

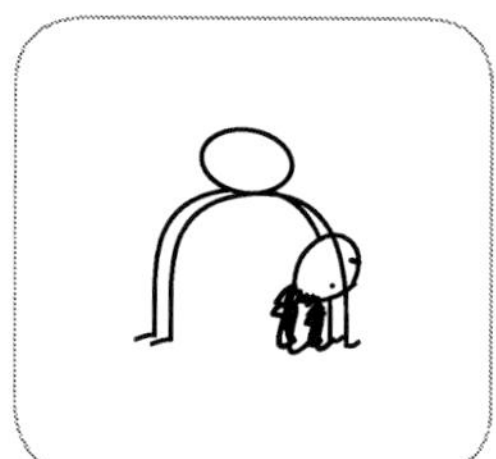

Urdhva Dhanurasana
(upward facing
bow pose)

MISCELLANEOUS

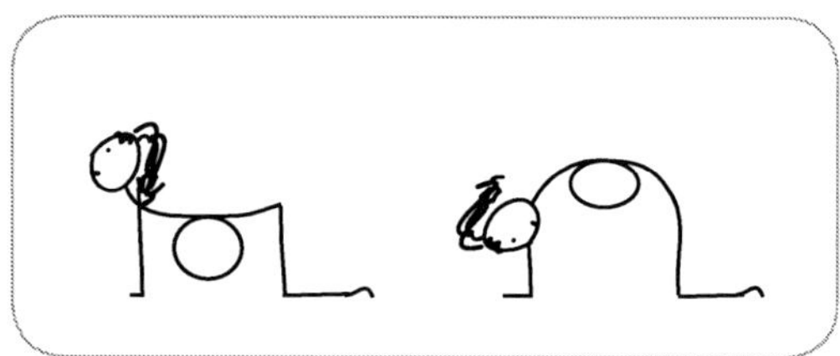

Cat/Cow Pelvic Tilts

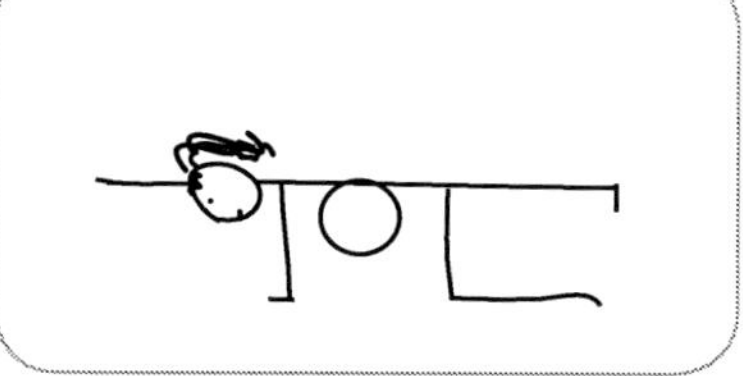

All Fours Variations
(balancing opposite arm/leg)

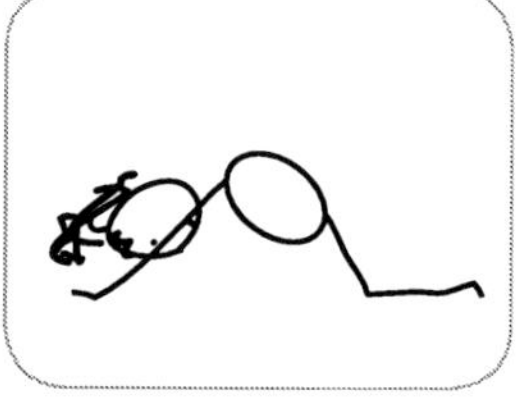

Adho Mukha Svanasana Prep
(quarter dog)

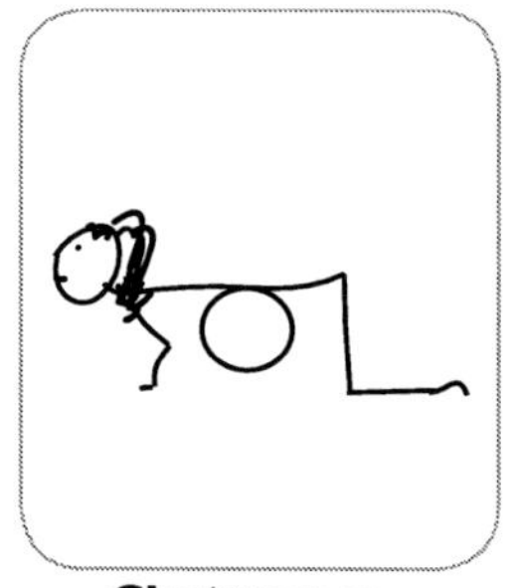

Chaturanga Push-ups
(four-limbed staff pose)

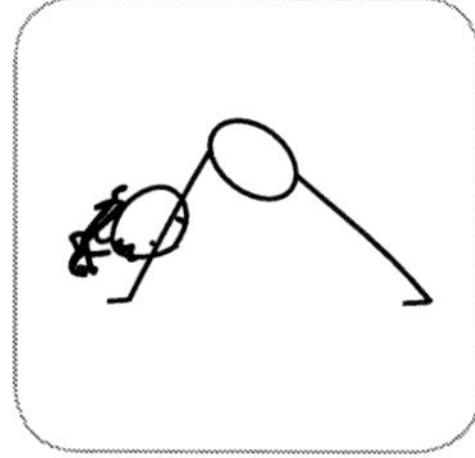

Adho Mukha Svanasana
(down dog)

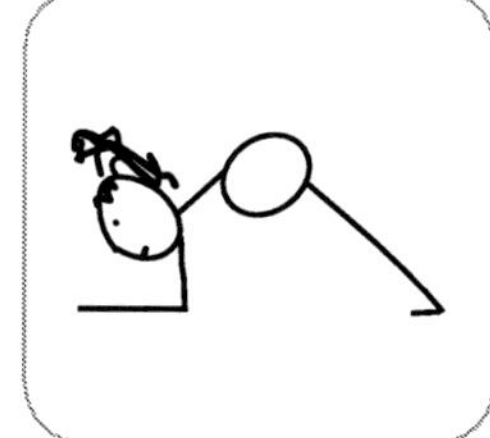

Pinca Mayurasana Prep
(dolphin)

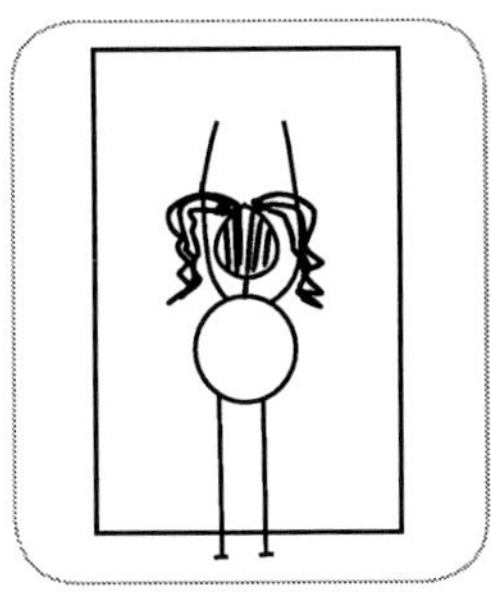

**Shower Pose
at Wall**

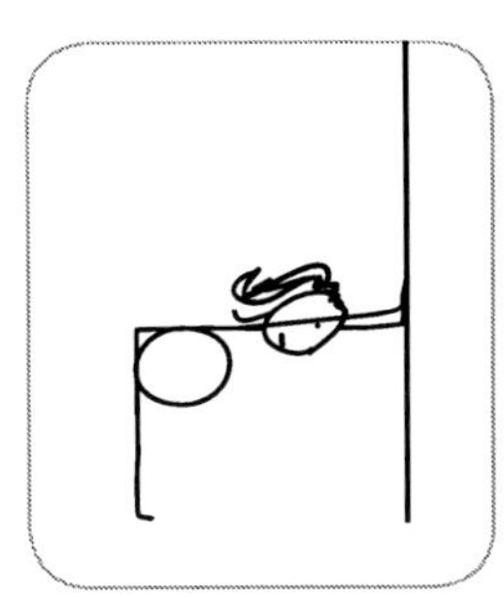

L-Pose

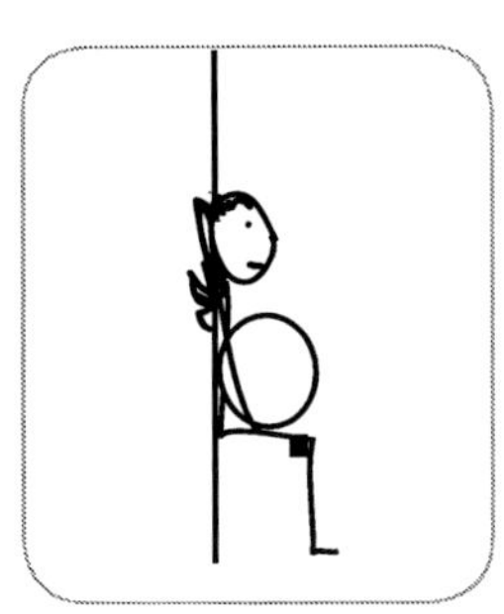

Wall Squat

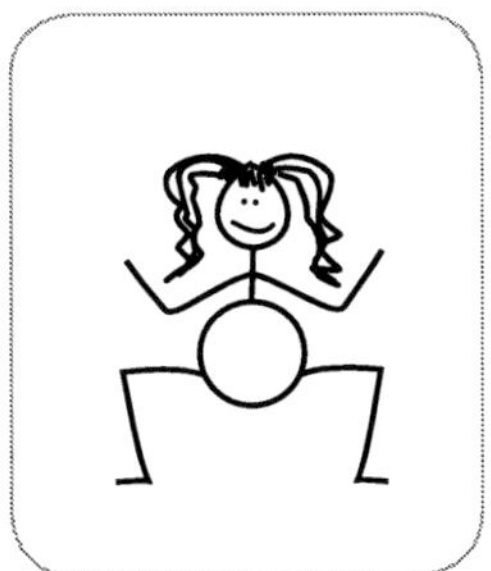

Goddess Pose

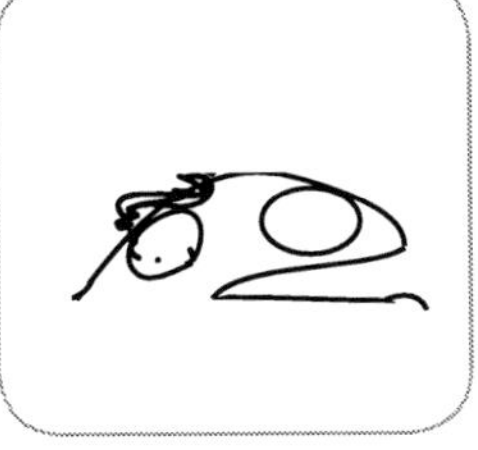

Balasana
(child's pose)

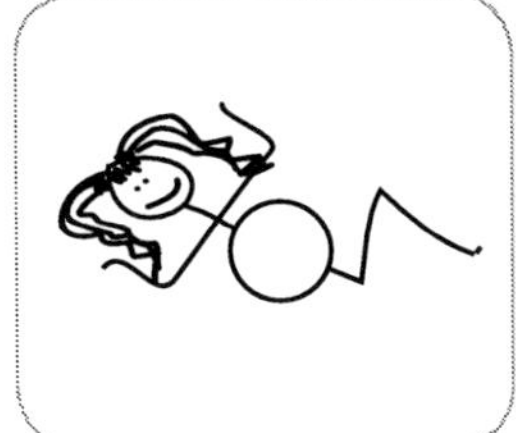

Supine Twist

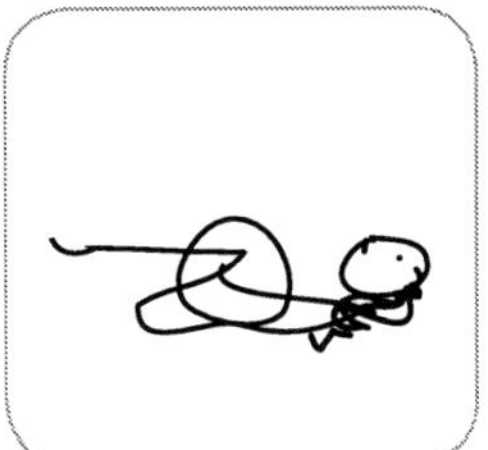

Supta Balasana
(reclined child's pose)

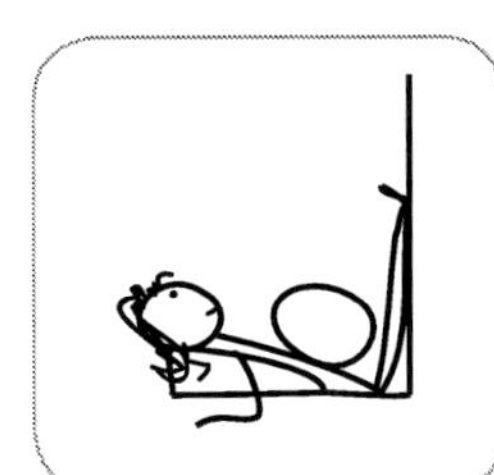

Viparita Karani
(legs-up-the-wall pose)

RESTORATIVES

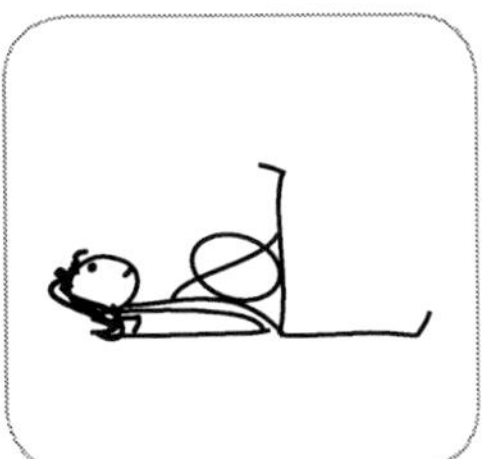

**Supta
Padangusthasana**
(reclined thigh-rooting
yoga pose)

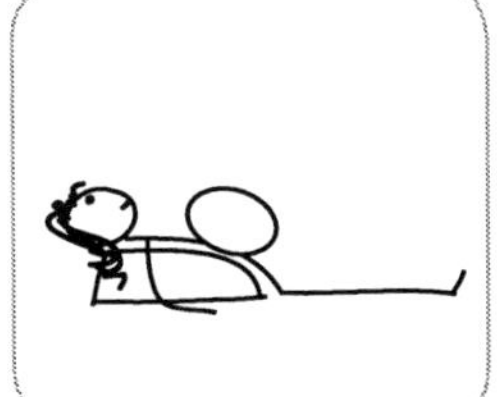

**Savasana
with Bolster**
(supported corpse pose)

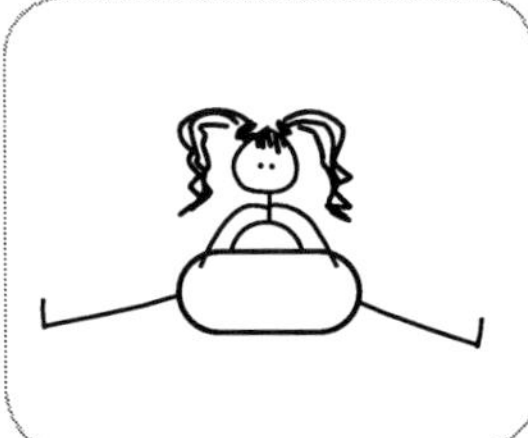

**Upavista Konasana using
Several Bolsters**
(supported wide-angle
forward bend pose)

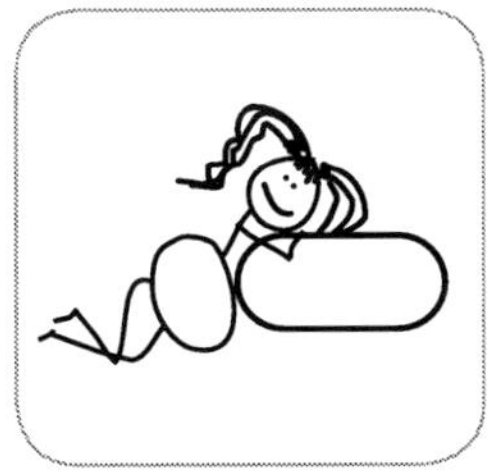

**Reclining Gentle Twists
with Bolster**

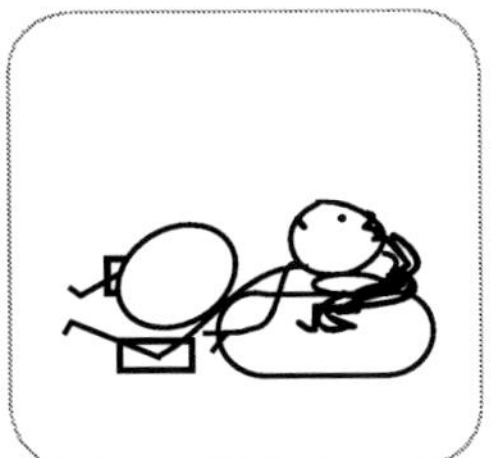

**Supported Supta
Baddha Konasana**
(reclined cobbler's pose)

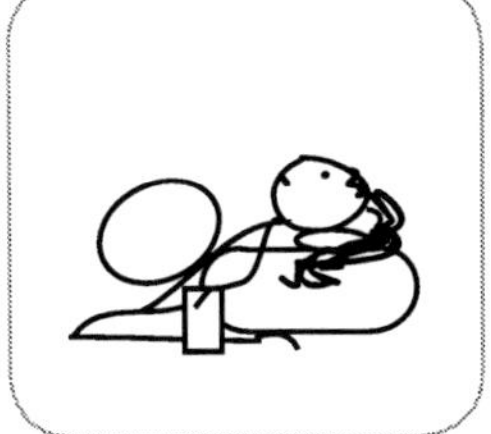

**Supported Supta
Virasana**
(reclined hero pose)

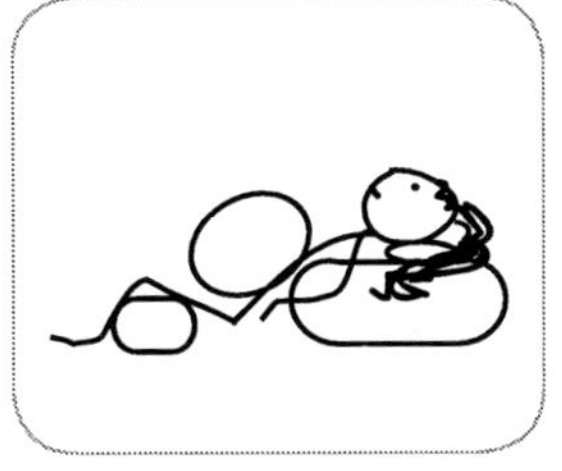

**Supported
Reclining Pose**

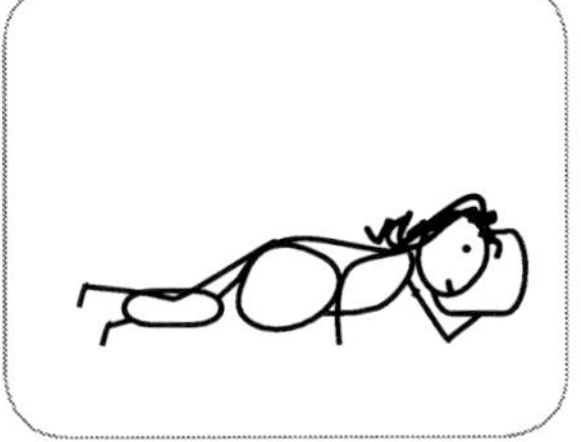

**Supported Savasana
on Left Side**
(reclined corpse pose)

ADDITIONAL RESOURCES

SUGGESTED READING LIST

Angier, Natalie. Woman : An Intimate Geography. Houghton Mifflin Harcourt Publishing Company, 1999.

Arms, Suzanne. *Immaculate Deception II: Myth, Magic & Birth*. Celestial Arts, 1994.

Balaskas, Janet. *Active Birth: The New Approach to Giving Birth Naturally*. The Harvard Common Press, 1992.

Balaskas, Janet. *Preparing for Birth with Yoga: Empowering and Effective Exercise for Pregnancy and Childbirth*. Thorsons, 2003.

Balaskas, Janet and Yehudi Gordon. *The Encyclopedia of Pregnancy and Birth: A Complete Self Help Guide to Active Birth and Early Parenthood, Including an A-Z of Modern Obstetrics*. Little, Brown Book Group, 1989.

Bradley, Robert. *Husband-Coached Childbirth: The Bradley Method of Natural Childbirth*. Bantam, 2008.

Buckley, Sarah. *Gentle Birth, Gentle Mothering*. Celestial Arts, 2009.

Calais-Germain, Blandine. *The Female Pelvis: Anatomy and Exercises*. Eastland Press Inc., 2003.

England, Pam and Rob Horowitz, Ph.D. *Birthing from Within: An Extra-Ordinary Guide to Childbirth Preparation*. Partera Press, 1998.

Fawcett, Margaret. *Aromatherapy for Pregnancy and Childbirth*. Element Books, 1993.

Gaskin, Ina May. *Ina May's Guide to Childbirth*. Bantam, 2003.

Gerber, Magda. *Dear Parent: Caring for Infants with Respect*. Resources for Infant Educators, 2003.

Gordon, Jay. *Listening to Your Baby: A New Approach to Parenting Your Newborn*. The Berkley Publishing Group, 2002.

Harris, A. Christine, Ph.D. *The Pregnancy Journal: A Day-to-Day Guide to a Healthy and Happy Pregnancy*. Chronicle Books, 2005.

Heller, Sharon, Ph.D. *The Vital Touch: How Intimate Contact With Your Baby Leads to Happier, Healthier Development*. Holt Paperbacks, 1997.

Herrera, Isa. *Ending Female Pelvic Pain: A Woman's Manual*. Duplex Publishing, 2014.

Khalsa, Gurmukh Kaur. *Bountiful, Beautiful, Blissful: Experience the Natural Power of Pregnancy and Birth with Kundalini Yoga and Meditation.* St Martin's Griffin, 2004.

Lasater, Judith Ph.D. *Relax and Renew: Restful Yoga for Stressful Times.* Rodmell Press, 1995.

Leboyer, Frederick. *Birth Without Violence.* Healing Arts Press, 2009.

Mayo Clinic. *Mayo Clinic Complete Book of Pregnancy and Baby's First Year.* William Morrow, 1994.

McCall, Timothy. *Yoga as Medicine: The Yogic Prescription for Health and Healing.* Bantam, 2007.

Mongan, Marie F. *HypnoBirthing, The Mongan Method: A Natural Approach to a Safe, Easier, More Comfortable Birthing.* Health Communications, Inc., 2005.

Newman, Dr. Jack & Pitman, Teresa. *Dr. Jack Newman's Guide to Breastfeeding.* Pinter & Martin Ltd., 2015.

Pearce, Joseph Chilton. *Magical Child.* Plume, 1992.

Romm, Aviva Jill. *The Natural Pregnancy Book: Herbs, Nutrition, and other Holistic Choices.* The Crown Publishing Group, 2003

Rost, Cecile. Relieving Pelvic Pain During and After Pregnancy. Hunter House Inc., Publishers, 1998.

Sears, Martha R.N. and William Sears M.D. *The Baby Book: Everything You Need to Know About Your Baby from Birth to Age Two.* Little, Brown and Company, 2003.

Sears, Martha R.N., William Sears M.D. and Linda Hughey Holt. *The Pregnancy Book.* Little, Brown & Company, 1997.

Simkin, Penny. *The Birth Partner: Everything You Need to Know to Help a Woman Through Childbirth.* Harvard Common Press, 2007.

Small, Meredith F. *Our Babies, Ourselves: How Biology and Culture Shape the Way We Parent.* Anchor, 1999.

Stein, Amy. Heal Pelvic Pain. McGraw-Hill Books, 2009.

Verny, Thomas M.D. and John Kelly. *The Secret Life of the Unborn Child: How You Can Prepare Your Baby for a Happy, Healthy Life.* Dell, 1982.

Weed, Susan. *Wise Woman Herbal: The Childbearing Year.* Ash Tree Publishing, 1985.

ONLINE RESOURCES

Birth:

babyfriendlyusa.org

birthingthefuture.com

birthintobeing.com

birthspsychology.com

birthworks.org/site/primal-health-research.html

childbirthconnection.org

choicesinchildbirth.org

fromwombtoworld.com

healing-arts.org/mehl-madrona/mmepidural.htm

holisticmoms.com

lovedelivers.org

mothering.com

normalbirth.org

ovu-tec.com/care.htm

pushedbirth.com

sciencebasedbirth.com

Breastfeeding — for more information or difficulty:

llli.org (La Leche League)

kellymom.com

Breech presentation — and for information about optimal fetal positioning:

spinningbabies.com

Cesarean — information on c-sections:

ican-online.org

Circumcision

nocirc.org

Doula — to learn more or locate one in your area:

dona.org

fromwombtoworld.com

Essential oils:

originalswissaromatics.com

oshadhiusa.com

floracopeia.com

Online magazines:

fitpregnancy.com

mothering.com

pregnancymagazine.com

Parenting — from conception through the childhood years:

askdrsears.com

drjaygordon.com

Postpartum/ Pelvic Floor Health:

postpartum.net

pelvichealthsolutions.ca

Preconception:

babycenter.com

foresight-preconception.org.uk

Pregnancy information:

americanpregnancy.org

cordblood.com

verywell.com

pregnancyweekly.com

prenatalkula.com

motherandchildhealth.com

socalbirth.com

thebump.com

Prenatal nutrition:

mayoclinic.com

Prenatal yoga:

digpregnancy.com

prenatal yoga video(2000) - Sue Elkind /Crunch Yoga Mama — amazon.com

Vaccinations:

nvic.org

Waterbirths:

waterbirthsolutions.com

"And then the time came,
when the risk it took to remain tight in a bud,
was more painful than
the risk it took to bloom"
— *Anais Nin*

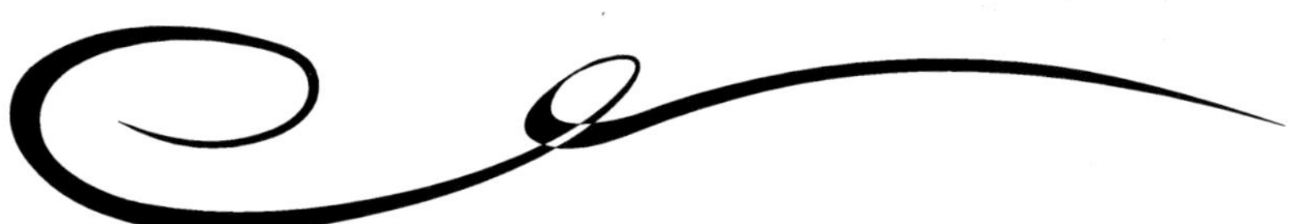

I would like to thank my beautiful family, Naime, Luca and Milo, for their illuminating presence in my life. There would be no book without them. I would also like to thank the following friends and family for their inspiration over the years which has helped me see this book through from conception to birth: Mary & Mort Elkind, Anna Verwaal, Douglas Brooks, Mae Sakharov, Barbara Benedict, Dana Covello, Gina Rubel, Denise Orloff, Allison Lorenzen, Clare Brown, Kim Kemper, Nancy Tarlow, and Sianna Sherman.